AF680351

SALINLUNAS

SALINLUNAS

NATURAL PRODUCTS & PHARMACOGNOSY

BRIAN POLLO

Copyright © 2025 ni Brian Pollo

All rights reserved.

First edition

Manila, Philippines

Para sa University of the Philippines

College of Pharmacy

Table of Contents

INTRODUCTION: NATURE'S LABORATORY

If one were to wander through a dense forest, the casual observer might see only greenery, light dappling through leaves, and the quiet motion of branches in the wind. Yet for those attuned to subtler truths, the forest is a vast laboratory, a workshop of alchemy and strategy, in which plants have spent millions of years perfecting molecules that protect, defend, attract, and sometimes seduce. Every leaf, root, and resinous exudate is an experiment in survival, conducted with a sophistication that would put any human laboratory to shame.

The plant kingdom, in essence, is a chemist's workshop. Its reagents are sunlight, water, and minerals; its catalysts are enzymes, evolving over eons to produce molecules of astonishing diversity and potency. Alkaloids, terpenoids, phenolics, flavonoids, and polyketides are the products of this natural laboratory, each with a defined role, each with a story of evolutionary purpose. These are not abstractions: they are chemical characters in dramas of survival and interaction, and humans, almost incidentally, have become participants in these narratives.

Historically, the connection between humans and these molecular actors is as old as civilization itself. Traditional healers observed patterns: the willow bark that relieved fever, the foxglove leaf that steadied the heart, the cinchona bark that quelled the shivers of malaria. Ethnobotanical anecdotes abound, tales of healers tasting, smelling, and observing plants, slowly decoding which offered relief and which demanded caution. These empirical observations, recorded in texts or preserved orally, form the foundation of pharmacognosy. They reveal a truth both humbling and inspiring: human knowledge of medicine is deeply indebted to the intelligence embedded in the natural world.

Modern science, of course, has taken this understanding further, dissecting the hidden machinery that produces these compounds. Biosynthetic pathways reveal why one plant produces morphine while another produces atropine; why a leaf is bitter to deter herbivores and simultaneously antimicrobial; why some flowers exude volatile terpenoids that repel predators and attract pollinators. Understanding these pathways is not mere academic curiosity. It is a gateway to innovation. By tracing the enzymatic steps, identifying precursors, and mapping regulation, scientists have learned to extract, synthesize, or even engineer these molecules for human benefit.

Take, for instance, the pathway to morphine in *Papaver somniferum*. Starting from the amino acid tyrosine, a sequence of enzyme-mediated steps (*e.g.*, hydroxylations, methylations, cyclizations) transforms a simple precursor into a molecule capable of profound physiological effect. Each step is a small story of chemical ingenuity, a narrative of evolution that balances defense, metabolic cost, and ecological advantage. Such molecular storytelling is everywhere in plants; it is what distinguishes pharmacognosy from mere herbalism, what elevates it from tradition into science.

Biosynthesis also teaches humility. Plants produce these molecules not for us, but for themselves, to defend, to attract, to survive. We are, in a sense, fortunate eavesdroppers, reading messages that were never intended for human consumption. Yet in this fortunate circumstance lies both opportunity and responsibility. The compounds we isolate are potent; they must be understood, handled, and applied with care. Misuse can harm, overharvesting can threaten ecosystems, and ignorance can reduce a miracle to a mere curiosity.

As this book will explore, the molecular drama of plants is vast. In **Part I**, we will meet the characters (*i.e.,* the alkaloids, terpenoids, phenolics, flavonoids, and polyketides) each with evolutionary purpose, each with a story of discovery. In **Part II**, we will witness the evolutionary drama itself: the selective pressures, symbioses, and molecular arms races that shape the chemical arsenal. **Part III** will bring us into human hands, detailing how folk remedies became modern medicines, and how biosynthetic insights guided discovery and innovation. Finally, **Part IV** will peer into the future, examining synthetic biology, conservation, and ethical considerations.

Ultimately, pharmacognosy is more than a catalog of molecules and pathways. It is a narrative of survival, adaptation, and human curiosity. It is a reminder that the molecules coursing through a leaf or resin are not inert; they are living stories, chemical expressions of strategy, history, and interaction. To study them is to participate in a dialogue spanning species and centuries, a dialogue in which humans have learned to read the hidden language of nature.

In turning these pages, the reader will learn to see plants not merely as background scenery, but as laboratories, laboratories where evolution has conducted meticulous experiments in chemistry. Every alkaloid, every flavonoid, every terpenoid is an experiment in survival. And, in the hands of careful scientists, an experiment in healing. To understand pharmacognosy is to step into this laboratory, to witness the elegance of molecular design, and to appreciate the profound intelligence encoded in the natural world.

SALINLUNAS

PART I

UGAT: MOLECULAR ESSENCE OF PHARMACOGNOSY

CHAPTER 1: ALKALOIDS ARE NEUROCHEMISTS

If plants are laboratories, alkaloids are among their most sophisticated experiments. These nitrogen-containing compounds are not casual byproducts of metabolism; they are purpose-built, evolutionary tools, designed to defend, repel, and occasionally enchant. In every bitter leaf, every pungent root, alkaloids lie in wait, shaping the interactions between plants and the world around them. Yet, for humans, they are more than defenses. They are medicines, agents that act upon our nervous systems, our hearts, our minds.

The story begins in the soil and sun, where plants evolved strategies to survive predation. Herbivores, insects, and microbes apply constant pressure, and in response, plants developed chemical sentinels: the alkaloids. Morphine (Figure 1), for instance, is a product of the opium poppy (*Papaver somniferum*), evolved to dissuade animals from consuming its delicate sap. The bitter taste, the numbing sensation, the toxicity at high doses, these are all part of a sophisticated defense mechanism. Humans, over centuries, learned to taste, observe, and measure these effects, gradually transforming a deterrent into a healer.

Alkaloids are remarkably diverse in structure and function. They include simple molecules such as nicotine, complex polycyclic compounds like morphine, and quinoline derivatives exemplified by quinine. Their evolutionary purpose is equally varied: some target herbivore nervous systems, others disrupt microbial cell division, and yet others serve as allelopathic agents, inhibiting the growth of competing plants nearby. Each alkaloid is a story of chemical ingenuity shaped by selective pressure.

Understanding the biosynthesis of alkaloids reveals the precision with which evolution works. Most alkaloids derive from amino acids (*e.g.*, tyrosine, tryptophan, lysine, ornithine) through enzyme-catalyzed transformations. Consider morphine biosynthesis: tyrosine is first converted into L-DOPA, then through a series of methylations, hydroxylations, and cyclizations, the molecule assumes the characteristic pentacyclic structure that interacts so potently with opioid receptors. Each enzyme acts with exquisite specificity, guiding the transformation of a simple amino acid into a molecule capable of altering perception, relieving pain, or sedating.

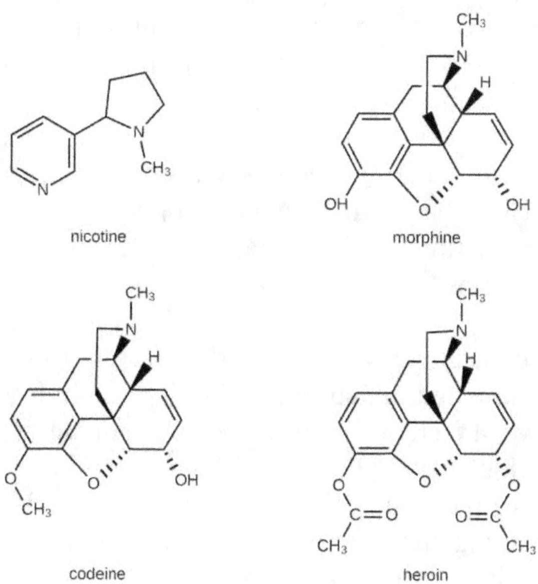

Figure 1. Alkaloids. OpenStax, CC BY 4.0 <https://creativecommons.org/licenses/by/4.0>, via Wikimedia Commons

Quinine, extracted from the bark of the cinchona tree, tells a similar story of evolutionary strategy and human ingenuity. Its biosynthesis begins with tryptophan and secologanin, converging in a condensation reaction catalyzed by strictosidine synthase. The resulting alkaloid is highly bitter, a deterrent to herbivores, and possesses antimalarial activity, which humans discovered empirically before understanding its chemical mechanism. The pathway is an elegant tapestry of reactions, each step a testament to evolutionary optimization: simple precursors giving rise to molecules capable of extraordinary biological effects.

Atropine, derived from *Atropa belladonna* (Figure 2), offers yet another glimpse into the intersection of plant defense and human medicine. Its role in deterring herbivory is clear: the tropane alkaloid acts as a neurotoxin, inhibiting muscarinic acetylcholine receptors and producing profound physiological effects. Yet humans, with careful dosing, have repurposed atropine as a life-saving agent: dilating pupils for ophthalmology, countering nerve agent poisoning, or treating bradycardia. Here, as in all of pharmacognosy, understanding the molecular action is inseparable from appreciating its evolutionary origin.

These compounds also reveal a remarkable story of convergent evolution. Across unrelated plant families, similar alkaloid structures have arisen independently, a chemical solution to recurring ecological challenges. Morphinan-like structures, quinoline derivatives, and tropane alkaloids appear in different lineages, reflecting the consistent pressures of herbivory and microbial attack. Nature, in this sense, is a master problem solver, repeatedly arriving at similar chemical solutions to analogous threats.

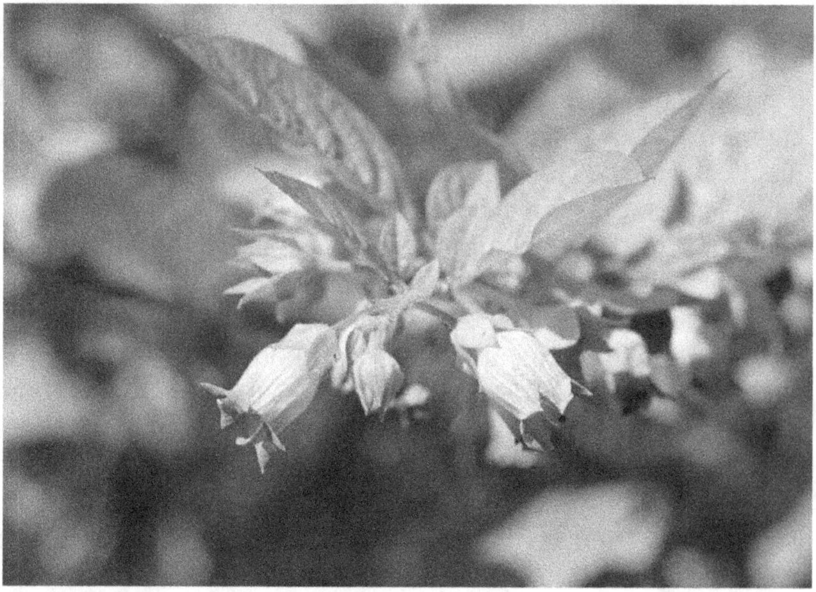

Figure 2. Atropa belladonna in the Botanischer Garten, Berlin-Dahlem._Krzysztof Ziarnek, Kenraiz, CC BY-SA 4.0 <https://creativecommons.org/licenses/by-sa/4.0>, via Wikimedia Commons

The human story interweaves with these natural narratives. Opium use dates back millennia, recorded in Sumerian texts and Egyptian papyri. Quinine saved countless lives during colonial campaigns against malaria, transforming history and geopolitics. Atropine, once feared as a poison, became a cornerstone of medicine. Each discovery reflects careful observation, patience, and a willingness to learn from the intelligence embedded in plant chemistry. Pharmacognosy, then, is not merely a catalog of molecules; it is a record of human curiosity responding to the wisdom of evolution.

Modern science, of course, extends these insights. By elucidating biosynthetic pathways, chemists and biologists have been able to replicate, modify, and optimize alkaloid production. Total synthesis of morphine in the laboratory, semi-synthesis of derivatives such as codeine and oxycodone, and microbial engineering to produce precursors at scale demonstrate the practical applications of understanding these pathways. Knowledge of enzymatic steps allows us to anticipate, design, and innovate, thus transforming natural compounds into tailored therapies without overexploiting the source plants.

Yet the narrative of alkaloids is not without caution. Potency is a double-edged sword. A molecule that heals in micrograms can harm in milligrams. Alkaloid toxicity, whether in ricinine, strychnine, or coniine, reminds us that pharmacognosy is both a science and an ethical practice. Understanding the chemical, evolutionary, and ecological context is essential to safe and effective application. It teaches restraint as much as curiosity, humility as much as admiration.

In teaching alkaloids, one might focus on tables and structures, reaction schemes, and receptor interactions, as Trease & Evans do with methodical clarity. Yet the narrative perspective—seeing molecules as agents in a survival drama—adds a dimension of understanding that pure data cannot provide. When a student traces the pathway from tyrosine to morphine, they are not merely memorizing reactions; they are witnessing an evolutionary strategy, a chemical dialogue with the environment, and a human story of observation, translation, and application.

The richness of this chapter lies also in its stories. The discovery of quinine, derived from the bark that indigenous Andean peoples (Figure 3) had long used, illustrates how traditional knowledge intersects with chemical analysis. Morphine, isolated by Sertürner in the early 19th century, marked a milestone in the purification and standardization of plant compounds, bridging folk use with modern pharmacology. Atropine's journey from deadly berry to clinical tool exemplifies the delicate balance of respect, experimentation, and insight. Each tale is a microcosm of the broader narrative: plants, humans, and molecules entwined in a dialogue spanning centuries.

Alkaloids remind us that nature is both generous and precise. The molecules produced are solutions to problems, answers to selective pressures, and, serendipitously, solutions to human ailments. Their study combines chemistry, biology, history, and philosophy: a molecule is never just a molecule; it is a strategy, a defense, a story. Pharmacognosy, in this light, becomes a lens through which we understand evolution, survival, and the interconnectedness of life.

In closing, to study alkaloids is to step into a theater of chemical drama. Each molecule is a character, each pathway a plotline, and every interaction with a human observer a chapter in an ongoing story. Morphine, quinine, and atropine are not merely drugs; they are survivors, evolved over millennia to face threats, now serving as allies in the human pursuit of health. By appreciating both their evolutionary origins and molecular sophistication, we gain not only knowledge but a profound sense of connection—to the natural world, to history, and to the intricate dance of chemistry and life.

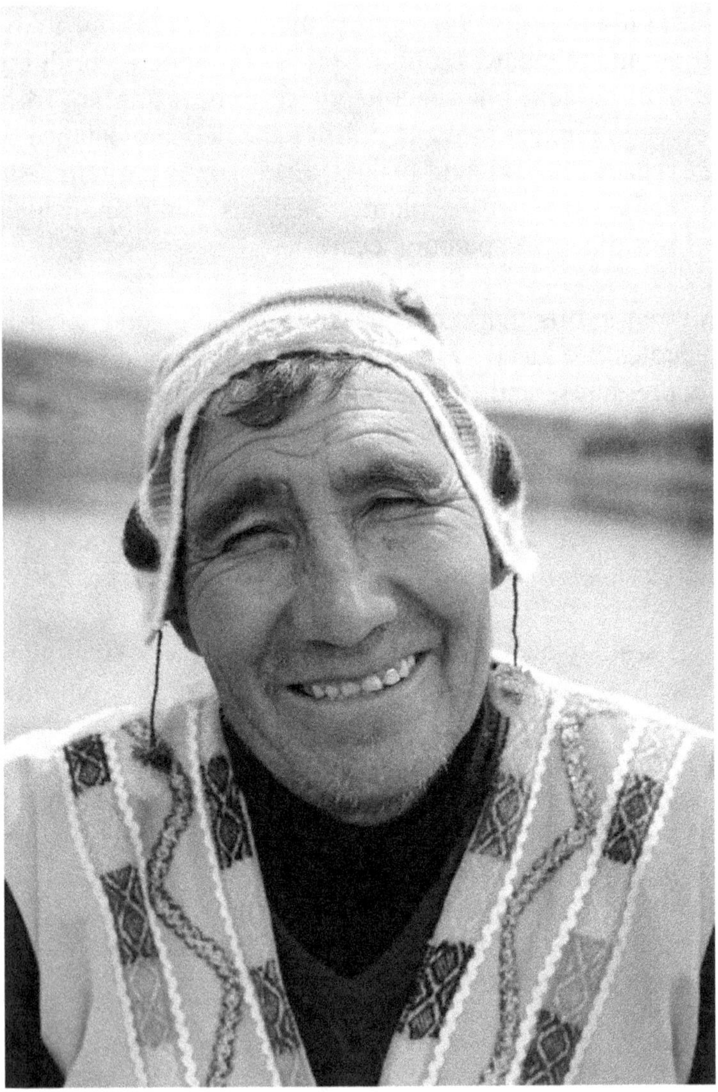

Figure 3. A Quechua man of the Andes mountains. Arenelii, CC BY-SA 4.0 <https://creativecommons.org/licenses/by-sa/4.0>, via Wikimedia Commons

CHAPTER 2: TERPENOIDS, MOLECULAR ARCHITECTS

If alkaloids are the secret agents of plant defense, terpenoids are the architects, dynamic, versatile, and astonishingly creative. Walk through a forest at dawn: the sharp scent of pine, the sweet aroma of citrus, the pungent whisper of eucalyptus in the wind. These fragrances are not accidents; they are chemical blueprints, carefully designed to communicate, protect, and sometimes seduce. Terpenoids are the molecules responsible, produced along pathways as ancient as the plants themselves, revealing the elegance of evolution as both chemist and strategist.

Terpenoids, sometimes called isoprenoids, are constructed from simple five-carbon units: isopentenyl pyrophosphate (IPP) and dimethylallyl pyrophosphate (DMAPP). These units, derived from the mevalonate (MVA) or methylerythritol phosphate (MEP) pathways, combine in modular fashion to form structures of remarkable diversity: monoterpenes, sesquiterpenes, diterpenes, triterpenes, and even the colossal tetraterpenes like carotenoids. The process is both disciplined and inventive: enzymes orchestrate condensation, cyclization, and oxidation with precision, yet the variety of products hints at an underlying creative freedom, a chemical artistry honed by evolution.

The ecological role of terpenoids is equally fascinating. Some serve as repellents, deterring herbivores with bitter, acrid, or irritating compounds. Others are attractants, signaling to pollinators with bright scents and volatile cues. Still others act as antimicrobial shields, protecting leaves and stems from fungal or bacterial invasion. In each case, the terpenoid is a tool of communication and survival, a molecule that mediates interactions between the plant and its world.

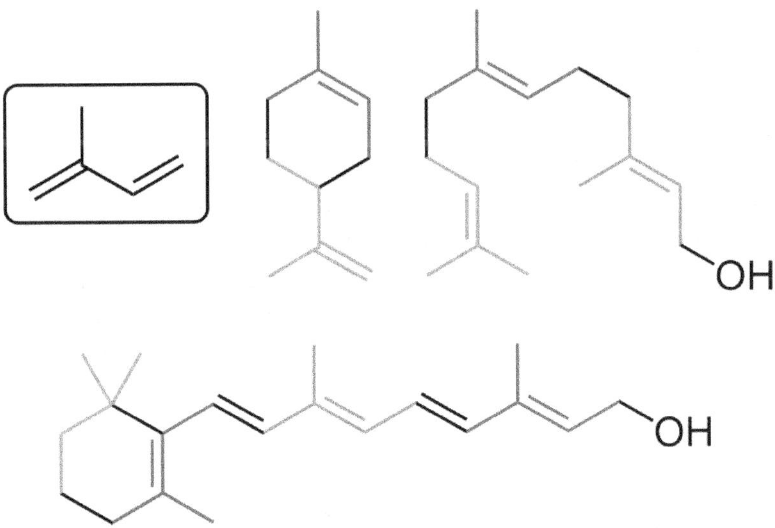

Figure 4. Assorted terpenoids (L-R: isoprene, limonene, farnesol, and retinol. Calvero., Public domain, via Wikimedia Commons

Consider paclitaxel, or Taxol, from the Pacific yew (*Taxus brevifolia*). In the wild, paclitaxel acts as a deterrent, preventing fungi from colonizing the tree's bark and leaves. Yet humans have recognized its extraordinary properties: paclitaxel stabilizes microtubules, preventing cell division, and became a cornerstone in cancer chemotherapy. The story of its discovery is emblematic of pharmacognosy: scientists guided by curiosity, ethnobotanical knowledge, and careful extraction revealed a molecule whose evolutionary purpose was survival, but whose human application is healing.

Artemisinin, derived from *Artemisia annua*, provides another example. In the plant, it is a chemical shield, reducing herbivore damage and resisting microbial infection. For humans, it became the spearhead against malaria, saving millions of lives. Its endoperoxide bridge (a subtle structural feature) is both an evolutionary triumph and a medicinal weapon (Figure 5). Here, the plant and the human converge: the molecule's design is optimized by nature, and its deployment is guided by science.

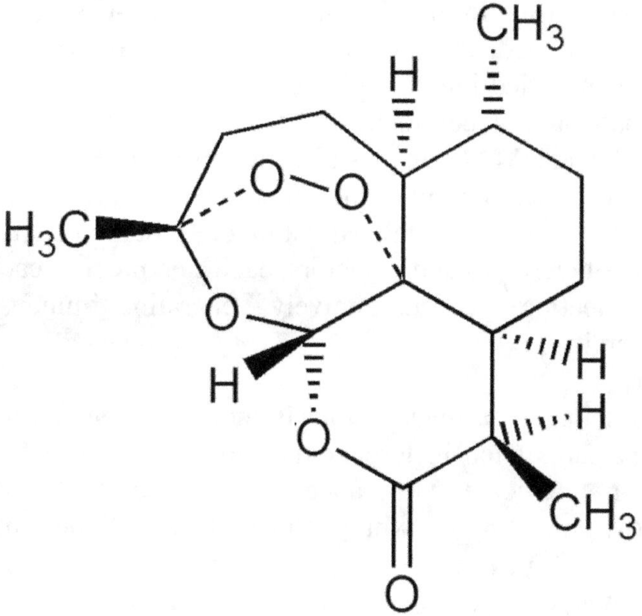

Figure 5. Artemisinin and its endoperoxide bridge. Mykhal at English Wikipedia, Public domain, via Wikimedia Commons

Terpenoids are not only defensive. They participate in intricate plant communication networks. Volatile monoterpenes can signal neighboring plants of herbivore attack, inducing the production of protective compounds in those neighbors. This chemical "language" transforms a forest into a network of sentient strategists, each individual responding to threats and opportunities in real time. Flavored and fragrant terpenoids also attract pollinators and seed dispersers, ensuring reproductive success. From an evolutionary standpoint, terpenoids are multifunctional tools. Defense, communication, and survival rolled into a single molecular package.

The biosynthetic pathways that generate these molecules are a marvel of enzymology. In the MVA pathway, acetyl-CoA units are assembled, reduced, and cyclized to form intermediates that can be further modified into complex diterpenes or triterpenes. In the MEP pathway, glyceraldehyde-3-phosphate and pyruvate give rise to IPP and DMAPP in plastids, supporting the synthesis of monoterpenes, carotenoids, and other critical molecules. These pathways, compartmentalized within cells, demonstrate a choreography of enzymes and cofactors, each step precise, each intermediate fleeting, yet cumulatively generating immense chemical diversity.

The human fascination with terpenoids is ancient. Essential oils, resins, and balsams (rich in terpenoids) have been prized for centuries for medicine, fragrance, and ritual. Modern pharmacology, guided by biosynthetic insights, has refined this knowledge, allowing extraction of specific terpenoids for use as drugs, flavorings, or bioactive compounds. Menthol, camphor, limonene, and carvone are examples of molecules that bridge tradition and modernity, embodying centuries of human observation and experimentation.

Mevalonate Pathway

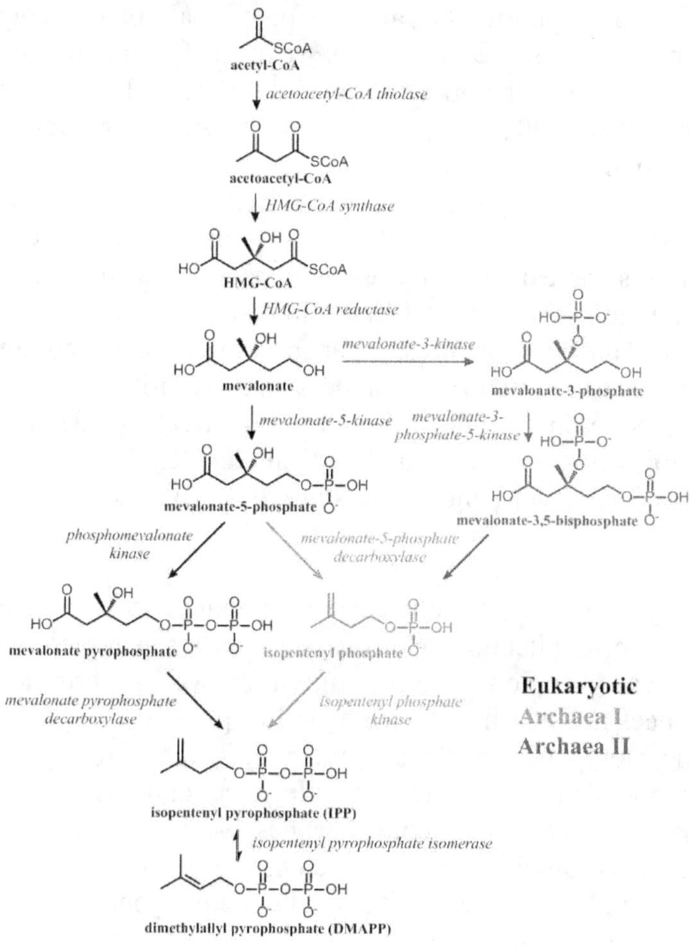

Figure 6. The mevalonate pathway. Uclasci1616, CC BY-SA 4.0 <https://creativecommons.org/licenses/by-sa/4.0>, via Wikimedia Commons

The narrative of terpenoids also carries caution. Many are potent; essential oils can irritate, damage tissues, or provoke allergic responses if misused. Yet their study exemplifies the balance of opportunity and respect that pharmacognosy demands. We observe, we isolate, we quantify, and only then do we translate into therapeutic application. The plant's strategy, refined over millennia, becomes a lesson in restraint and discernment.

Perhaps most striking is the evolutionary arms race that terpenoids reveal. Herbivores evolve resistance; pathogens adapt; plants respond by generating new terpenoid variants. Paclitaxel and artemisinin are snapshots in a dynamic continuum of chemical innovation, reminders that nature's laboratory is active, ongoing, and infinitely adaptive. Understanding terpenoids is not merely cataloging molecules. It is perceiving evolution in action, a molecular story of defense, adaptation, and survival.

In studying terpenoids, one must appreciate both structure and story. The architecture of a diterpene is inseparable from its ecological function; the configuration of a sesquiterpene influences its volatility, its scent, and its protective capacity. By tracing biosynthetic pathways, we gain insight into how plants solve chemical problems with elegance and efficiency. By observing the ecological consequences, we perceive the logic of chemical communication and defense. By understanding the human application, we witness the convergence of natural wisdom and scientific inquiry.

Ultimately, terpenoids are architects not only of molecules but of ecosystems. They construct invisible bridges between plants, insects, microbes, and humans. They shape behavior, survival, and adaptation. The study of terpenoids is simultaneously chemical, ecological, historical, and ethical; a reminder that the molecules we isolate are embedded in rich narratives of life.

As we leave this chapter, imagine walking through a garden or forest. Each scent, each resinous exudate, each flicker of fragrance in the wind is a story, a message, a strategic deployment of molecular ingenuity. Terpenoids are not merely compounds; they are active participants in the drama of survival, communicating, defending, and evolving. To study them is to witness nature's architecture in motion: a blend of creativity, utility, and resilience that humbles even the most accomplished human chemist.

CHAPTER 3: PHENOLICS AND FLAVONOIDS, SOLAR SHIELDS

Sunlight, in its generosity, bathes the world in warmth and illumination. Yet for the plant, light is both gift and hazard. Ultraviolet radiation can damage DNA, oxidize membranes, and provoke stress responses. How, then, do rooted organisms, unable to flee, endure the daily onslaught of photons? The answer lies in phenolics and flavonoids—molecules that act as the plant's solar shields, absorbing, reflecting, and quenching energy, while simultaneously participating in defense, signaling, and survival.

Phenolics, a broad class of compounds characterized by aromatic rings bearing hydroxyl groups, are ubiquitous in the plant kingdom. Flavonoids, a subclass of polyphenolics, are particularly remarkable for their structural diversity and multifunctionality. They absorb ultraviolet light, chelate reactive oxygen species, and mediate interactions with pollinators, pathogens, and herbivores. In essence, flavonoids are the molecular diplomats of the plant: protective yet communicative, defensive yet attractive.

Biosynthesis begins with the shikimate pathway, an evolutionary innovation that converts simple carbohydrates into aromatic amino acids such as phenylalanine and tyrosine. Phenylalanine, via the action of phenylalanine ammonia-lyase (PAL), gives rise to cinnamic acid, which serves as a precursor for an enormous array of phenolic compounds. Through hydroxylation, methylation, and glycosylation, the plant generates flavonoids, tannins, lignins, and other secondary metabolites—each tailored to a specific ecological purpose.

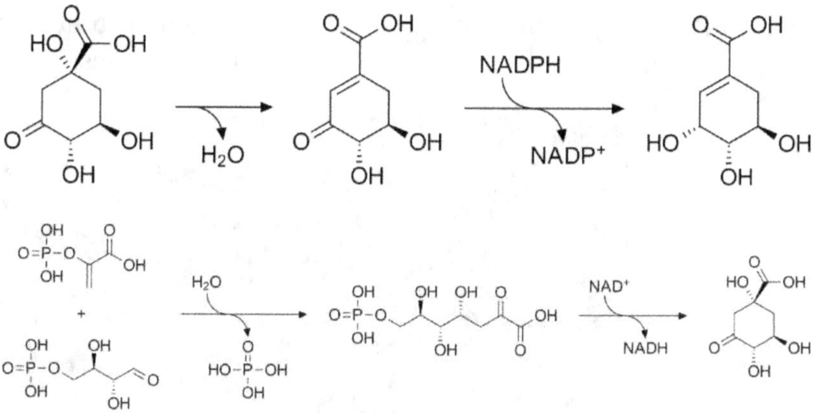

Figure 7. The shikimate pathway. Public domain.

Consider the anthocyanins, the pigments responsible for red, purple, and blue hues in flowers and fruits. While their visual allure attracts pollinators and seed dispersers, anthocyanins simultaneously protect tissues from UV damage and oxidative stress. In the leaves of high-altitude or sun-exposed plants, anthocyanins form a protective layer, absorbing potentially harmful radiation while allowing photosynthesis to proceed. Here, chemistry and ecology intersect: a single class of molecules achieves multiple objectives, a molecular compromise honed by evolution.

Flavonoids also function as antioxidants, neutralizing free radicals generated by light and metabolic activity. Reactive oxygen species, if unchecked, can damage lipids, proteins, and nucleic acids, compromising cellular integrity. Flavonoids donate electrons to these radicals, stabilizing them and preventing cellular damage. In human health, the same properties are leveraged for their anti-inflammatory, cardioprotective, and anticancer effects. Quercetin, kaempferol, and catechins, common dietary flavonoids, demonstrate the continuity of protective chemistry from plants to humans.

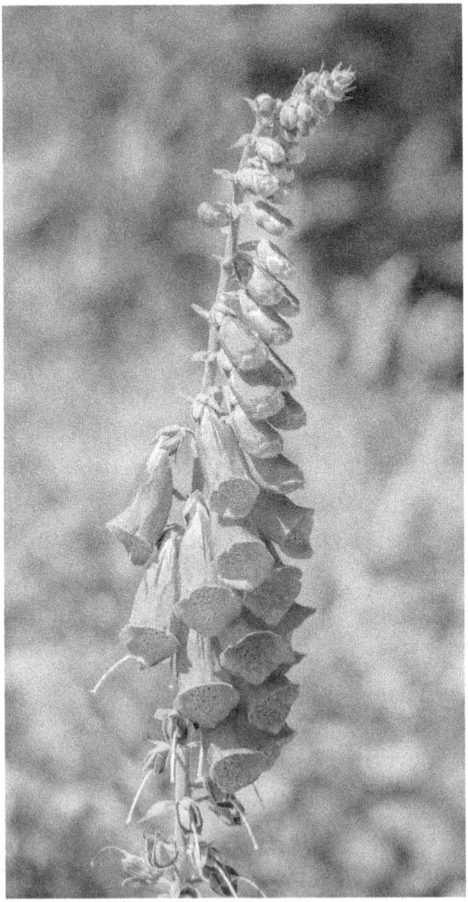

Figure 8. Digitalis purpurea. By H. Zell - Own work, CC BY-SA 3.0, https://commons.wikimedia.org/w/index.php?curid=93262087

Phenolics play an equally vital role in structural integrity and defense. Lignins, polymers of phenolic alcohols, reinforce cell walls, making stems rigid and resistant to microbial invasion. Tannins, bitter and astringent, deter herbivory by binding proteins and reducing digestibility. The evolutionary logic is clear: molecules that protect the plant from light damage, oxidative stress, pathogens, and grazers are retained, diversified, and optimized. Humans, observing these effects, have translated them into medicines, nutraceuticals, and dietary interventions.

Historical anecdotes illuminate this duality of protection and utility. Digitalis, a flavonoid-containing compound derived from *Digitalis purpurea* (Figure 8), stabilizes cardiac rhythm in humans while serving as a defense against herbivores. Willow bark, rich in phenolic salicylates, relieved human pain and fever long before the molecular mechanism of aspirin was understood. These stories exemplify the convergence of evolutionary design and human application, a theme recurring throughout pharmacognosy.

The complexity of flavonoid biosynthesis is both fascinating and instructive. Enzymes such as chalcone synthase, chalcone isomerase, and flavanone 3-hydroxylase guide the formation of diverse flavonoid structures (Figure 9). Methyltransferases, glycosyltransferases, and acyltransferases further modify these compounds, tailoring solubility, stability, and reactivity. In doing so, plants create a chemical palette of thousands of flavonoids, each with subtle differences in absorption spectra, antioxidant potential, and biological activity. For the pharmacognosist, mapping these pathways is akin to understanding the schematics of an elaborate architectural project, where form, function, and context are inseparable.

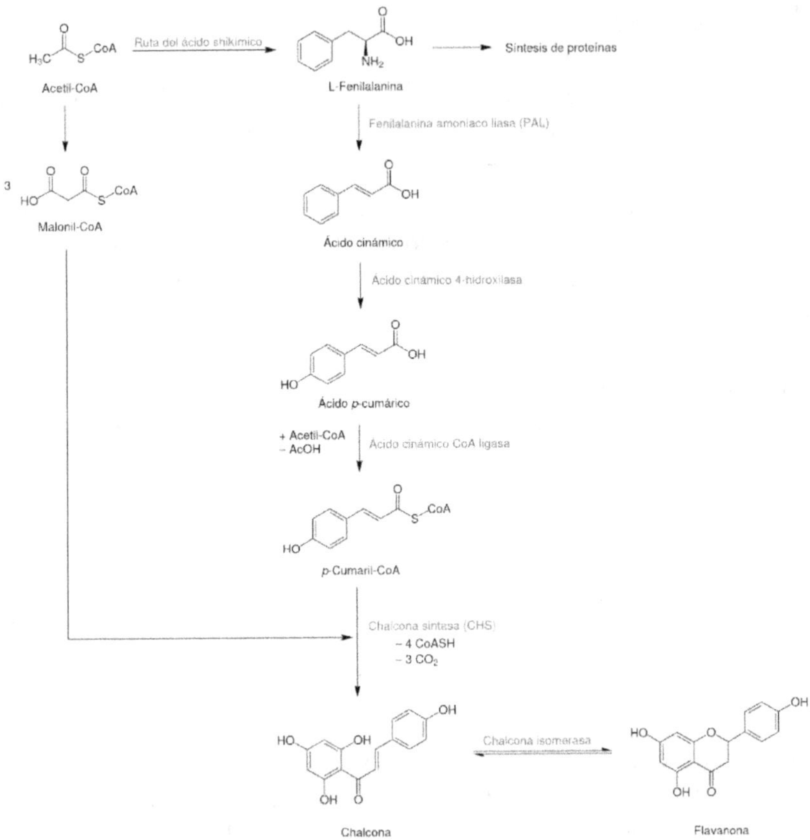

Figure 9. Biosynthesis of flavonoids. ChemSim, Public domain, via Wikimedia Commons

Flavonoids are also key players in signaling networks. They mediate symbiotic interactions with nitrogen-fixing bacteria, influencing root nodule formation. They attract pollinators through pigmentation, odor, and taste. They signal to neighboring plants, priming defense mechanisms against impending herbivore attack. These molecules are, in effect, both armor and messenger, protecting the plant while communicating its status to allies and adversaries alike.

Humans have learned to harness flavonoids with subtlety. Modern extraction methods (*e.g.,* maceration, Soxhlet extraction, and chromatographic separation) allow isolation of specific compounds for pharmacological use. Structural elucidation through spectroscopy and mass spectrometry reveals their molecular architecture, enabling synthetic modification and bioactivity optimization. The flavonoids that defend leaves from UV light now stabilize human cells against oxidative stress, demonstrating a profound continuity of chemical purpose across kingdoms.

Yet the story of phenolics is also one of restraint. Potency, context, and dosage matter. Overconsumption can be toxic, interact with other drugs, or alter nutrient absorption. The careful observation that guided ancient herbalists continues to be essential in modern pharmacognosy: molecules are powerful, but their application demands respect, knowledge, and precision.

Ecologically, flavonoids illustrate the ongoing evolutionary dialogue between plants and their environment. Sunlight, herbivores, pathogens, and microbial partners act as selective pressures, shaping flavonoid diversity. Plants in high-UV environments produce anthocyanins and flavonols in greater quantities. Herbivory induces specific flavonoid synthesis. Microbial symbionts influence the phenolic profile of roots and leaves. The molecules are adaptive responses, fine-tuned to ecological challenges, yet simultaneously useful to humans as medicines.

From a narrative perspective, flavonoids are characters in a story of light, stress, and survival. They embody protection, communication, and resilience. They teach the pharmacognosist to read chemical signals as stories: each pigment, each antioxidant, each signaling molecule is a paragraph in the ongoing narrative of life, evolution, and interaction. To study flavonoids is to witness the strategies by which plants negotiate survival under relentless environmental pressure, and to see how humans have learned to translate those strategies into healing.

As the sun falls behind the horizon, casting long shadows over leaves and flowers, one might pause to reflect on the elegance of this molecular theater. Phenolics and flavonoids, invisible yet pervasive, perform their roles without fanfare, absorbing energy, quenching radicals, signaling to friends and foes alike. They are, in every sense, the solar shields of life. Molecules that guard, communicate, and endure. And in studying them, we not only understand chemistry; we witness evolution, ecology, and human ingenuity converging in a single, radiant narrative.

CHAPTER 4: POLYKETIDES, EVOLUTION'S MODULAR DESIGNS

If alkaloids are secret agents and terpenoids are architects, then polyketides are the master builders of molecular diversity. They are modular, versatile, and ingeniously adaptive. In the microbial world, these compounds are often the first line of chemical offense, weapons honed through evolutionary trial and error to inhibit competitors, destroy invaders, or manipulate ecological niches. For humans, they have become some of the most potent medicines ever discovered: antibiotics, anticancer agents, immunosuppressants, and cholesterol-lowering drugs.

Polyketides are constructed via a process that is almost mechanical in its precision: iterative condensation of simple acyl-CoA units, guided by large enzymatic complexes called polyketide synthases (PKSs). Each module in the synthase acts as a station on an assembly line, adding, modifying, or cyclizing a building block to create intricate molecular architectures. This modularity is the genius of polyketide evolution: by rearranging modules, nature can generate enormous chemical diversity from relatively simple starting materials. It is an evolutionary strategy of efficiency, flexibility, and adaptability.

Consider erythromycin, produced by *Saccharopolyspora erythraea*. Its 14-membered macrolactone ring, decorated with sugars, is assembled step by step by a type I modular PKS. Each module carries a defined function (*e.g.,* chain elongation, reduction, dehydration, or cyclization) and the product is a precise, biologically active molecule capable of inhibiting bacterial protein synthesis. Evolution has honed these enzymes with such specificity that even minor alterations in module sequence can dramatically alter the final product's activity, demonstrating both the fragility and sophistication of nature's chemical engineering.

The evolutionary purpose of polyketides is evident in microbial ecology. Bacteria and fungi coexist in competitive environments, where space and nutrients are scarce. Producing polyketides allows these organisms to inhibit competitors, defend territories, and survive environmental pressures. Penicillin, produced by *Penicillium* species, exemplifies this strategy: the β-lactam ring inhibits bacterial cell wall synthesis, giving the mold a decisive advantage in crowded ecological niches. What began as a microbial survival tactic became, centuries later, a human lifesaving drug.

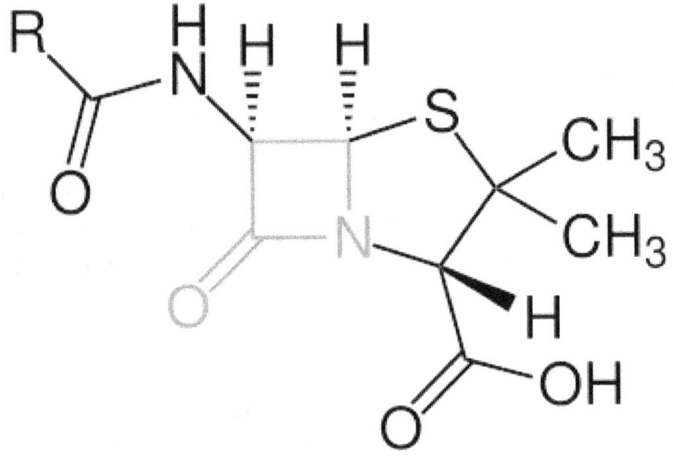

Figure 10. Penicillin general structure, showing the beta-lactam ring. Jü, CC BY-SA 4.0 <https://creativecommons.org/licenses/by-sa/4.0>, via Wikimedia Commons

Polyketides also illustrate convergent chemical evolution. Despite the diversity of organisms that produce them (*i.e.,* fungi, bacteria, plants) the principles of modular assembly recur, suggesting that evolution repeatedly discovers the power of iterative synthesis. Lovastatin, the first naturally occurring statin, inhibits HMG-CoA reductase, controlling cholesterol biosynthesis. Its structure, produced via a fungal polyketide pathway, mirrors the strategy seen in antibiotics: modular construction of a complex molecule with precise biological function. Evolution, in this sense, is a clever engineer, reusing patterns of chemical assembly to solve diverse ecological problems.

The human discovery story of polyketides is as dramatic as their molecular complexity. Penicillin's accidental discovery by Alexander Fleming in 1928 transformed medicine, turning previously fatal infections into treatable conditions. Erythromycin, discovered in soil actinomycetes, provided an alternative to penicillin for those allergic or resistant. These discoveries were not random. They emerged from careful observation, experimentation, and an understanding that microbes produce bioactive compounds as part of ecological strategy. By tracing these evolutionary designs, humans could co-opt microbial chemistry for therapeutic purposes.

Biosynthetically, polyketides are remarkable in their enzymatic precision. Type I PKSs operate as megasynthases, modular and programmable, whereas type II PKSs form multi-enzyme complexes that iteratively cyclize aromatic polyketides. Type III PKSs, simpler yet elegant, catalyze condensation reactions without carrier proteins, often generating plant polyketides. Each type exemplifies nature's ability to solve chemical design problems in distinct ways, demonstrating flexibility and innovation within the same overarching molecular logic.

Polyketides' structural diversity also underlies their pharmacological breadth. Macrolides (erythromycin, azithromycin) inhibit bacterial protein synthesis (Figure 11); tetracyclines disrupt ribosomal function; anthracyclines (doxorubicin) intercalate DNA, preventing cancer cell replication (Figure 12); epothilones stabilize microtubules, akin to paclitaxel. Across these applications, the common theme is modular construction. A chemical assembly line capable of producing molecules with complex, specific, and potent biological effects.

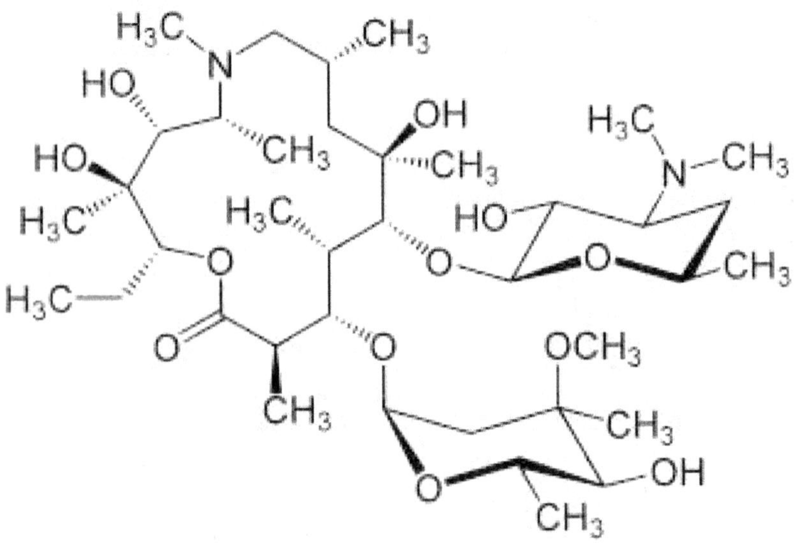

Figure 11. Azithromycin. Yikrazuul, Public domain, via Wikimedia Commons

Modern science has leveraged these insights to engineer polyketides. Synthetic biology allows swapping of PKS modules, tailoring products with altered pharmacokinetics, improved potency, or reduced toxicity. Semi-synthetic derivatives optimize natural molecules for human therapy, while total synthesis allows production independent of natural sources. Here, understanding biosynthetic logic is not mere curiosity. It is a tool for innovation, bridging natural evolution and human ingenuity.

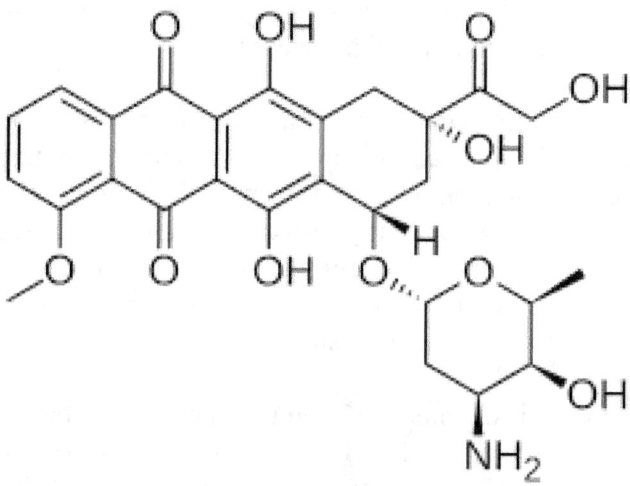

Figure 12. Doxorubicin. Fvasconcellos 23:30, 4 May 2007 (UTC), Public domain, via Wikimedia Commons

The detective story of polyketides also reveals the challenges of pharmacognosy. Molecules may be produced in minute quantities, embedded in complex matrices, or exist only under specific environmental conditions. Isolation, structural elucidation, and activity testing demand patience, skill, and careful observation. Yet these challenges are matched by the rewards: lifesaving antibiotics, anticancer agents, and drugs that alleviate chronic disease, all derived from microbial chemical warfare.

Ecologically, polyketides remind us that chemistry is a language of survival. Compounds evolve to solve immediate threat (*e.g.*, competing microbes, predation, environmental stress) but humans have learned to read and interpret this language, translating it into therapeutic action. The molecules are ancient strategists, refined over millennia, now collaborating with human intelligence to combat disease.

In narrative terms, polyketides are modular protagonists in a story of molecular adaptation. Each module contributes to character, function, and fate. Each enzymatic step is a clue in an evolutionary detective story, revealing how organisms solve chemical problems with ingenuity and precision. Humans, by deciphering these clues, become co-authors in an ongoing saga of survival, chemistry, and healing.

As we close this chapter, imagine the microscopic battleground: a mold colony spreading over a damp substrate, secreting penicillin into the surrounding medium; a soil bacterium producing erythromycin to outcompete neighbors. In each molecule, we perceive strategy, design, and foresight—chemical intelligence distilled into a structure that can, centuries later, save human lives. Polyketides, modular yet precise, are evolutionary triumphs, reminders that nature's laboratory is not only vast but endlessly inventive.

PART II

PAKIKIBAKA: STRUGGLE OF PLANTS IN CO-EVOLUTION

CHAPTER 5: CHEMICAL WARFARE OF PLANTS VERSUS PATHOGENS

In the quiet of a forest, an invisible war rages. Leaves glisten with morning dew, but each droplet may conceal the first strike of a microbial invader. Stems, roots, and flowers are battlegrounds, contested by viruses, bacteria, fungi, and herbivores alike. Plants, rooted and unable to flee, have evolved a chemical arsenal—an array of secondary metabolites that function as weapons, shields, and signals. This is the theater of chemical warfare, where survival is dictated not by brute strength, but by molecular ingenuity.

Imagine a leaf under attack by a pathogenic fungus. Within hours, the plant mobilizes defenses: flavonoids accumulate to quench oxidative stress, phenolics cross-link cell walls to create barriers, terpenoids volatilize to repel the invader or signal neighboring plants. Alkaloids and polyketides may be secreted to disrupt the metabolism of the pathogen. Each response is orchestrated with precision, reflecting millions of years of evolutionary fine-tuning. Every molecule tells a story of selective pressure, adaptation, and resilience.

This chemical arsenal is astonishingly diverse. Convergent evolution has produced similar defensive compounds in unrelated plant lineages. Phenolics appear in angiosperms and gymnosperms alike; terpenoids are ubiquitous from conifers to flowering herbs; alkaloids arise in poppies, nightshades, and legumes. The repeated emergence of similar chemical strategies underscores the universality of selective pressures—fungi attack, herbivores graze, and survival favors the clever chemist. Evolution, in this sense, is a relentless strategist, iteratively discovering solutions to recurrent ecological problems.

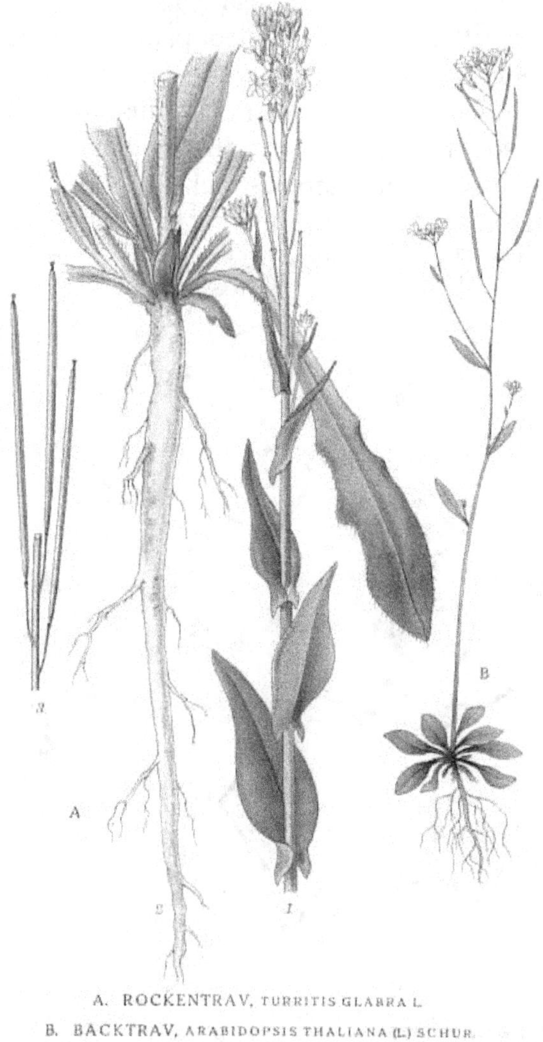

Figure 13. Arabidopsis thaliana. By Carl Axel Magnus Lindman - «Bilder ur Nordens Flora» Stockholm, Public Domain,

https://commons. wikimedia.org/w/index.php?curid=5969392

Pathogens themselves evolve. Virulence factors, effector proteins, and detoxifying enzymes counteract plant defenses. This sets the stage for an arms race, chemical against chemical, strategy against strategy. Plants that can detect pathogen attack early and mount a rapid secondary metabolite response survive; those that fail are culled. Over generations, this dynamic produces molecular sophistication: compounds that inhibit microbial enzymes, disrupt membranes, chelate essential metals, or induce programmed cell death in infected tissues. The battlefield is microscopic, but the stakes are survival.

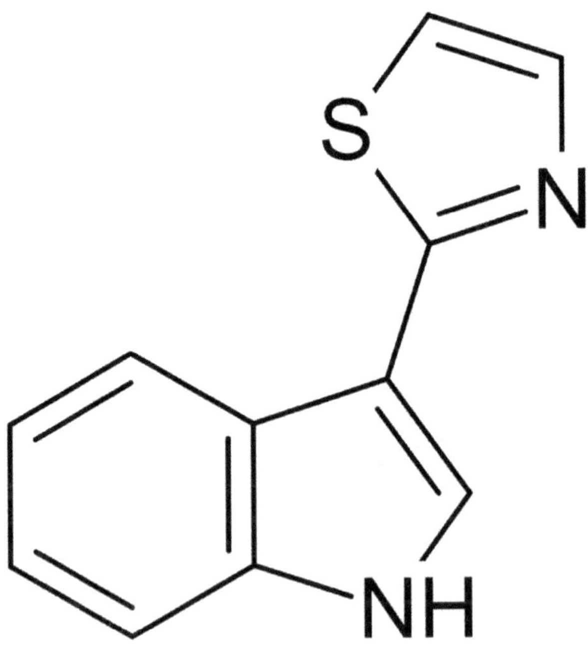

Figure 14. Camalexin. By Ed (Edgar181) - Own work, Public Domain, https://commons.wikimedia.org/w/index.php?curid=38485359

Consider phytoalexins, low-molecular-weight compounds synthesized de novo in response to infection. Camalexin, produced by *Arabidopsis thaliana* (Figure 13), is a sulfur-containing indole phytoalexin that inhibits fungal growth (Figure 14). Its synthesis is tightly regulated: upon pathogen recognition, specific enzymes convert tryptophan into camalexin via a series of hydroxylations, methylations, and cyclizations. This response is rapid, localized, and highly effective, a molecular counterstrike executed within hours. Humans studying these pathways have gleaned insights into plant immunity and potential applications in agriculture and medicine.

Another dramatic example is the role of terpenoid phytoanticipins, compounds present before attack but deployed selectively. Monoterpenes and sesquiterpenes in conifer resin (Figure 15), for instance, serve both as deterrents to herbivores and as antifungal agents. When bark beetles bore into trees, resin flows, rich in volatile terpenoids, suffocating larvae, inhibiting fungal growth, and signaling neighboring trees. This is not passive chemistry; it is active warfare, a chemical choreography of defense, deterrence, and communication.

Polyketides, too, participate in plant-pathogen interactions. Some serve as antifungal agents, disrupting cell wall synthesis or interfering with metabolic enzymes. Others act as signaling molecules, triggering systemic acquired resistance in distal tissues. These molecules are modular in design, enabling plants to rapidly evolve new variants to counter pathogen adaptation. The biosynthetic flexibility mirrors that seen in microbial polyketides: modularity allows innovation without starting from scratch, a strategy that evolution has perfected.

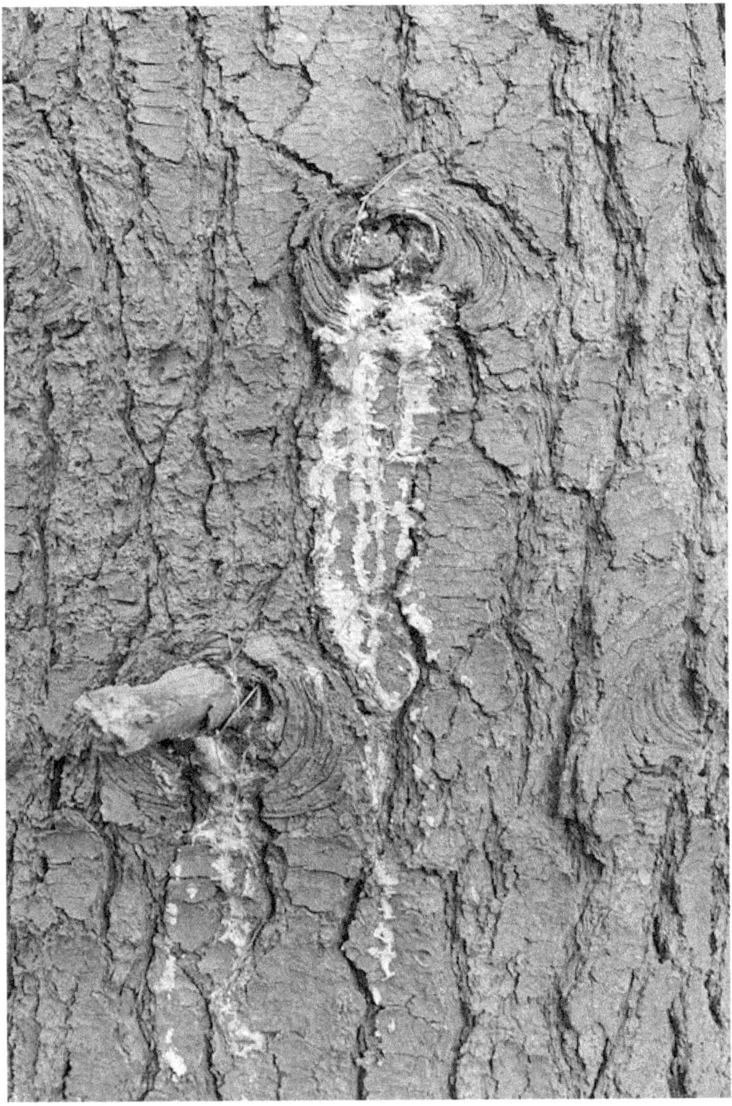

Figure 15. Conifer resin, rich in terpenoids. Ryan Hodnett, CC BY-SA 4.0 <https://creativecommons.org/licenses/by-sa/4.0>, via Wikimedia Commons

Humans, observing these chemical battles, have often appropriated the outcomes. Antibiotics like penicillin were originally microbial weapons in competitive soil environments. Alkaloids such as quinine were developed by plants to defend against herbivores, yet became humanity's defense against malaria. Understanding plant chemical defenses has therefore guided not only pharmacognosy but also agriculture, where phytoanticipins and phytoalexins inspire natural pesticide development.

The evolutionary narrative embedded in chemical warfare is compelling. Each compound represents a solution to a survival problem, and each structural variation is a response to selective pressure. Pathogens evolve resistance, herbivores adapt to toxins, and plants respond by producing new molecules or modifying existing ones. Over millions of years, this dialogue has produced the incredible chemical diversity we observe today. We see a library of solutions to ecological challenges, written in atoms and bonds.

This cinematic war is also spatial and temporal. Different tissues deploy different molecules; young leaves may have high concentrations of alkaloids to deter grazing, while mature leaves invest more in structural phenolics. Roots secrete flavonoids to shape microbial communities; flowers produce volatile terpenoids to attract pollinators while repelling herbivores. Timing is critical: rapid induction of phytoalexins can mean the difference between infection and survival. Plants, though rooted, are agile chemists, modulating chemistry with sophistication that rivals any human strategy.

Ecological interactions further complicate the drama. Symbiotic fungi or bacteria can enhance plant chemical defenses, producing metabolites in concert with the host. Conversely, some pathogens manipulate plant metabolism, redirecting resources away from defense. Each encounter is a story of negotiation, adaptation, and conflict. Each is a molecular dialogue unfolding in real time. By studying these interactions, pharmacognosists uncover principles that guide not only drug discovery but also ecosystem management and sustainable agriculture.

The human story intersects with this drama repeatedly. From traditional herbalists observing which plants resisted spoilage or insect attack, to modern scientists elucidating the biosynthetic pathways of antifungal alkaloids, we have learned to read the chemical narratives plants write. Every discovery—camalexin, paclitaxel, quinine—is a translation of evolutionary strategy into human utility. Yet the molecules themselves remain testament to the intelligence of natural selection: they were never produced for us, only co-opted by our curiosity, insight, and ingenuity.

In narrative terms, chemical warfare casts plants as tacticians, pathogens as challengers, and humans as informed observers. The drama is dynamic, continuous, and instructive. Molecules are deployed, countermeasures enacted, and adaptations iterated over generations. The forest, the soil, and the garden are all theaters of this invisible conflict, where survival favors those capable of chemical foresight.

As we step back from this battlefield, the lesson is clear: secondary metabolites are not mere curiosities; they are the currency of life. Each alkaloid, flavonoid, terpenoid, and polyketide is a tactical solution to a biological problem, a response to selective pressure, a story of survival encoded in chemical structure. To study them is to witness evolution's strategies in molecular detail, to appreciate the elegance and brutality of natural selection, and to recognize the profound intelligence inherent in the living world.

The forest, once perceived as serene, becomes alive with strategy, conflict, and innovation. Leaves, stems, and roots are weapons, shields, and messengers. Microbes, insects, and herbivores are adversaries, each shaping the evolution of plant chemistry. And humans, curious and observant, enter the scene as readers, translators, and beneficiaries of a chemical saga millions of years in the making. In this theater, every molecule matters, every pathway tells a story, and every interaction is a lesson in survival, adaptation, and ingenuity.

CHAPTER 6: SYMBIOSIS AND CO-EVOLUTION

Life, at its core, is relational. No organism exists in isolation. Every leaf, root, or flower is embedded within a network of unseen collaborators. Plants, remarkable as they are, owe much of their chemical prowess not solely to their own genomes, but to the microbial partners with which they co-evolve. Symbiosis (mutualism, commensalism, and even the subtle tug-of-war of parasitism) shapes the secondary metabolites that define pharmacognosy. In these intimate alliances, chemical innovation emerges, pathways are shared, and evolution accelerates.

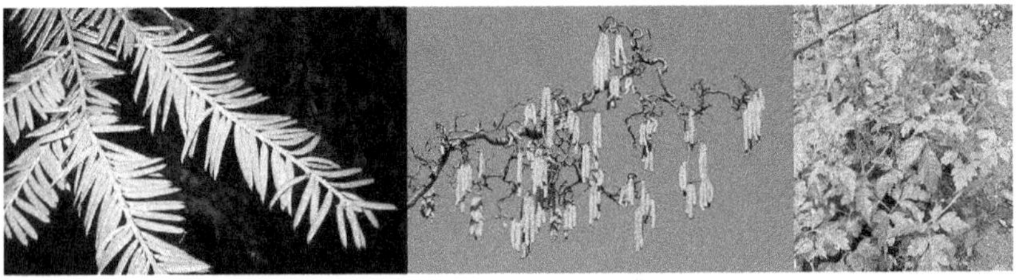

Figure 16. Taxol containing plants. L-R: hazelnut, Taxus, Cardiospermum halicacabum. Walter Siegmund (talk) Schnobby H. Zell, CC BY-SA 3.0 <https://creativecommons.org/licenses/by-sa/3.0>, via Wikimedia Commons

Endophytic fungi and bacteria are perhaps the most intriguing contributors. Hidden within plant tissues, often without causing symptoms, these microbes produce a remarkable array of bioactive compounds. Some polyketides, terpenoids, and alkaloids originally attributed to the plant are in fact microbial products, or at least the result of combined biosynthetic effort. The discovery of *Taxomyces andreanae*, an endophytic fungus producing paclitaxel (Taxol), revolutionized our understanding of natural product origin: what had been considered a plant molecule was partially microbial, revealing a hidden layer of chemical collaboration.

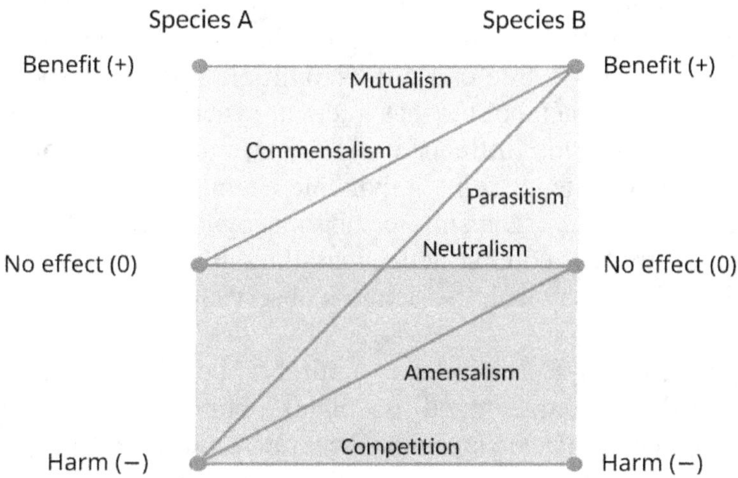

Figure 17. Diagram of symbiotic relationships. Ian Alexander, CC BY-SA 4.0 <https://creativecommons.org/licenses/by-sa/4.0>, via Wikimedia Commons

Horizontal gene transfer adds another dimension. Genes responsible for secondary metabolite biosynthesis can move between plant-associated microbes, enabling rapid acquisition of biosynthetic capabilities. In some cases, plants themselves appear to have incorporated microbial genes, creating hybrid pathways that neither partner could produce alone. Consider the production of indole alkaloids: some endophytes supply precursors or enzymes, while the plant completes the pathway, yielding a potent defensive molecule. Evolution, in this sense, is not linear; it is a network of chemical exchange, innovation, and co-adaptation.

Symbiosis also shapes chemical specificity (Figure 17). Endophytes may produce molecules tailored to their plant host, suppressing pathogens or modulating herbivore behavior. The leaves of a single tree can harbor multiple microbial species, each secreting metabolites that interact, synergize, or compete. These interactions influence the plant's overall secondary metabolite profile, creating a dynamic chemical mosaic unique to that individual organism. For pharmacognosists, this implies that bioactivity is context-dependent: the same species grown in sterile culture may lack the richness observed in nature.

Some endophytes produce entirely novel compounds, previously uncharacterized in plants. For example, fungal endophytes of *Artemisia annua* generate unique sesquiterpene derivatives that complement the plant's artemisinin. Similarly, bacterial symbionts in the roots of medicinal legumes secrete flavonoid-like molecules, modulating plant development and defense. These discoveries suggest that many classical plant drugs may be products of microbial-plant co-evolution, blurring the boundaries between "plant" and "microbe" chemistry.

Co-evolution extends beyond chemical production to ecological interactions. Plants may selectively recruit microbes through root exudates, sugars, or signaling molecules, fostering communities that enhance resistance to disease or environmental stress. Microbes, in turn, evolve mechanisms to persist, avoid plant defenses, or manipulate host metabolism. This is not passive cohabitation; it is an active negotiation, a molecular dialogue mediated by secondary metabolites. Each party benefits, but each is also under selective pressure to maintain its own fitness.

This dialogue can have striking consequences for human medicine. Consider epiphytic bacteria that influence the alkaloid content of *Catharanthus roseus* (Figure 18), the source of vincristine and vinblastine. Variations in microbial composition directly affect the yield of these anticancer compounds. Understanding the co-evolutionary dynamics between plant and microbe allows pharmacognosists to optimize production, either through microbial inoculation, tissue culture, or metabolic engineering. Here, ecology informs chemistry, and collaboration informs discovery.

Symbiotic co-evolution also offers insights into the evolution of chemical novelty. Recombination of biosynthetic modules across microbial and plant genomes generates molecules with structural features never previously observed. Hybrid polyketides, alkaloid derivatives, and flavonoid conjugates arise from the mingling of enzymatic pathways across species boundaries. Evolution, in this sense, is a laboratory of shared intelligence: the molecule is both artifact and messenger, encoding the history of collaboration, conflict, and adaptation.

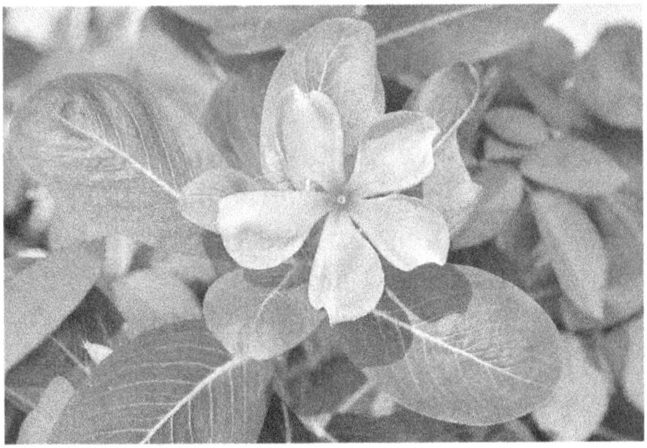

Figure 18. Catharanthus roseus. Photo: Joydeep / Wikimedia Commons

Consider the example of pyrrolizidine alkaloids in certain grass species. Recent studies suggest that endophytic bacteria contribute enzymes that alter precursor availability, enhancing the diversity of alkaloid structures. This symbiosis allows plants to generate a broader spectrum of defensive molecules than they could alone, creating a chemical repertoire that improves survival against herbivores and pathogens. Humans, again, benefit: these unique alkaloids inspire drug discovery programs targeting cancer, infection, and neurological disorders.

Beyond direct biosynthesis, symbiosis shapes plant signaling and developmental pathways. Flavonoid production, induced by microbial cues, may regulate root architecture, leaf morphology, or flowering time. Terpenoid emission can be modulated by endophytic interactions, altering volatile-mediated communication with pollinators and herbivores. Chemical networks are therefore multi-layered: a molecule may defend, signal, and coordinate development simultaneously, reflecting co-evolved complexity.

The human story intersects with these discoveries in profound ways. Techniques like metagenomics, metabolomics, and synthetic biology allow researchers to dissect these networks, revealing hidden contributors to known drugs. Endophytes once considered incidental are now recognized as vital collaborators, expanding the potential of pharmacognosy. By mimicking or harnessing these symbiotic interactions, scientists can enhance yield, discover new compounds, or even engineer entirely novel biosynthetic pathways.

Ethically, the study of symbiosis also emphasizes conservation. Loss of microbial diversity through deforestation, monoculture, or environmental stress may irreversibly alter the chemical landscape of medicinal plants. Protecting both plant and microbial partners ensures the continued availability of natural products and preserves the evolutionary processes that generate chemical innovation. The pharmacognosist is therefore both a chemist and a steward, observing nature's laboratory while safeguarding its capacity to innovate.

Narratively, symbiosis reframes the story of pharmacognosy. Rather than a tale of individual plants defending themselves, it becomes a story of networks: chemical alliances, enzymatic collaborations, and evolutionary negotiation. Microbes, once invisible players, are now co-protagonists, shaping the molecules we study, the drugs we develop, and the ecological strategies we admire. Every secondary metabolite is no longer solely a product of the plant, but a shared narrative of co-evolution, adaptation, and innovation.

In closing, the study of symbiosis and co-evolution invites us to reconsider agency in nature. Plants are not lone chemists; they are collaborators, negotiators, and network participants.

Microbes are not passive passengers; they are chemical engineers, partners in biosynthesis, and drivers of novelty. Together, they create molecules of astonishing diversity and potency. Molecules that humans can translate into medicines, insights, and inspiration.

Walking through a forest, one might imagine the invisible conversations taking place: fungal hyphae secreting modulatory compounds, bacterial colonies supplying precursors, plant cells orchestrating enzymatic assembly. Every molecule is a word in this conversation, every pathway a sentence, every bioactive compound a story of millions of years of shared evolution. Pharmacognosy, in this light, becomes the study of dialogue (chemical, ecological, and historical), and a testament to the intelligence inherent in life's collaborative design.

CHAPTER 7: THE MOLECULAR ARMS RACE

In the intricate tapestry of life, plants and pathogens engage in a relentless evolutionary battle. This dynamic interaction, often referred to as the "molecular arms race," is characterized by the continuous development of chemical defenses by plants and the counter-adaptations by pathogens. At the heart of this conflict lies the production of secondary metabolites—diverse chemical compounds that serve as potent weapons in the plant's defense arsenal.

Plants, rooted in place and unable to flee from threats, have evolved a sophisticated array of chemical defenses to deter herbivores and pathogens. These secondary metabolites, including alkaloids, terpenoids, phenolics, and glucosinolates, are not essential for basic metabolic processes but play crucial roles in defense and signaling.

- **Alkaloids**: Nitrogen-containing compounds like nicotine and morphine deter herbivores and pathogens through toxicity or deterrence.
- **Terpenoids**: Volatile compounds such as limonene and menthol serve as repellents or toxic agents against a wide range of organisms.
- **Phenolics**: Flavonoids and tannins can inhibit pathogen growth and reduce herbivory by affecting digestion.
- **Glucosinolates**: Found in cruciferous plants, these compounds break down into toxic products upon tissue damage, deterring herbivores.

The biosynthesis of these compounds is often induced by environmental stressors or pathogen attack, highlighting their role in adaptive responses to biotic threats.

In response to plant defenses, pathogens have developed an array of strategies (*i.e.*, counter-adaptations) to overcome chemical barriers. These include the secretion of effector proteins that suppress plant immune responses, the evolution of detoxifying enzymes that neutralize plant toxins, and the ability to alter host metabolism to facilitate infection.

For instance, certain bacterial pathogens produce enzymes that degrade plant-produced antimicrobial compounds, while some fungi have evolved mechanisms to secrete toxins that suppress plant defense gene expression. These countermeasures exemplify the ongoing evolutionary pressure exerted by plant defenses.

This co-evolutionary arms race is not a static phenomenon but a dynamic interplay where each party continuously adapts to the other's strategies. As plants evolve new chemical defenses, pathogens respond with counter-adaptations, leading to an ever-escalating cycle of innovation and counter-innovation.

An illustrative example is the interaction between *Arabidopsis thaliana* and the fungal pathogen *Botrytis cinerea* (Figure 19). Upon infection, *Arabidopsis* activates the biosynthesis of camalexin, a sulfur-containing phytoalexin with antimicrobial properties. In turn, *Botrytis* has developed mechanisms to degrade camalexin, allowing it to persist and proliferate within the host tissue. This reciprocal adaptation underscores the dynamic nature of the plant-pathogen arms race. Interestingly, despite this arms race, *Arabidopsis* and *Botrytis* have been found to engage in horizontal gene transfer as well Figure 19)!

Understanding the molecular basis of this arms race has profound implications for agriculture and medicine. By elucidating the mechanisms underlying plant chemical defenses and pathogen counter-adaptations, researchers can develop strategies to enhance crop resistance to diseases and pests. Additionally, insights gained from these interactions can inform the discovery of novel antimicrobial agents, as many plant-derived compounds exhibit potent activity against human pathogens.

For example, the discovery of the plant-derived compound paclitaxel, used in cancer therapy, was a direct result of studying plant secondary metabolites. Similarly, the exploration of plant-derived alkaloids has led to the development of drugs for various ailments, including hypertension and malaria.

The molecular arms race between plants and pathogens is a testament to the power of evolutionary processes in shaping the chemical landscape of life. Through the continuous development and refinement of chemical defenses and counter-defenses, both plants and pathogens contribute to the dynamic equilibrium of ecosystems. As we deepen our understanding of these interactions, we unlock the potential to harness nature's ingenuity in addressing challenges in agriculture and medicine.

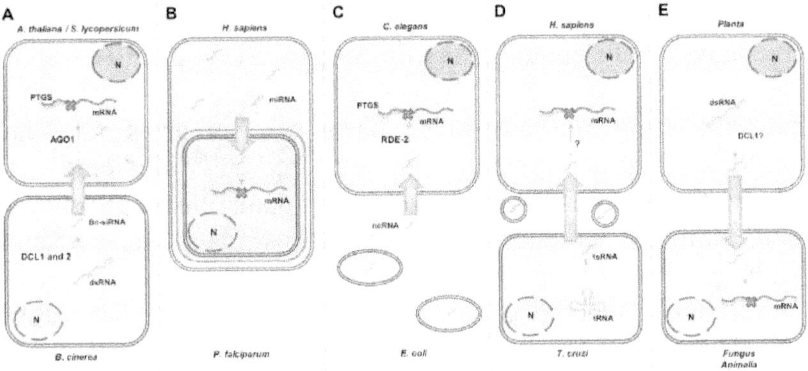

Figure 19. Botrytis cinerea can transfer Bc-siRNA to its host. This process has been shown to be dependent on AGO1 in the host, Arabidopsis thaliana and on both Dcl1 and 2 in Botrytis cinerea. B, Human miRNAs can be translocated to the malaria-parasite, P. falciparum, where they interfere with translation. C, The nematode C. elegans has been shown to take up E. coli-produced ncRNAs that subsequently influence their foraging behavior. This is dependent on the C. elegans protein RDE-2, that is essential for RNAi. D, The Chagas disease-causing parasite, T cruzi, produces tRNA-derived sRNAs (tsRNAs) that are exported from the cell in vesicles. These vesicles are shown to increase infectability of host cells, suggesting this might be caused by the tsRNAs. This has not been shown directly though. E, The expression of sRNA-generating constructs to silence genes in pathogens, or other closely associated species, has now been demonstrated for many species combinations. This process is suggested to be dependent on Dcl1, since Dcl2, 3, and 4 seem to be dispensable to induce silencing by an Arabidopsis-expressed hairpin in the insect, Helicoverpa armigera. Knip M, Constantin M, Thordal-Christensen H, CC BY 4.0 <https://creativecommons.org/licenses/by/4.0>, via Wikimedia Commons

PART III

PAMANA: OUR NATURAL PRODUCTS HERITAGE

CHAPTER 8: FROM FOLK REMEDIES TO MODERN MEDICINE

Long before the first chemistry textbooks, humans were observers of the living world, taking notes not with pens but with experience. They watched which leaves soothed wounds, which roots eased fever, and which flowers caused nausea or paralysis. Each observation was a hypothesis tested across seasons and generations, a dialogue with nature mediated by trial, error, and intuition. These early experiments, often couched in ritual and tradition, were not the crude practices one might imagine. They were sophisticated empirical studies grounded in careful observation of cause and effect.

Ethnopharmacology, the systematic study of traditional medicine, reveals a remarkable pattern: the plants used in folk remedies often contain secondary metabolites with proven biological activity. Willow bark, used for millennia to alleviate pain and fever, contains salicylates, precursors of modern aspirin. The Cinchona tree, once a secret of Andean healers, produces quinine, still used today to combat malaria. Morphine, extracted from poppy latex, was recognized long before its molecular mechanism was understood. What is striking is the convergence of human ingenuity and evolutionary strategy: plants evolved these chemicals as defenses, yet humans discovered their utility by careful trial and observation.

The process of turning folk remedies into modern medicine is itself a story of discovery layered upon discovery. It begins with extraction, the first act of separation in the laboratory of observation. Simple maceration or boiling isolates soluble compounds, revealing the bitter, aromatic, or acrid components that often hint at biological activity. Chromatography and crystallization refine this process, allowing isolation of pure molecules, while spectroscopic techniques (*e.g.*, NMR, mass spectrometry, and UV-Vis analysis) unveil the architecture of atoms. The transformation from leaf, root, or bark to chemical formula is a translation of nature's language into human terms.

Yet even this process owes a debt to evolutionary strategy. Secondary metabolites are not arbitrary; they are products of millions of years of selection for specific functions (*e.g.*, antifeedant, antioxidant, antimicrobial, or signaling molecules). Alkaloids like atropine evolved to deter herbivores, flavonoids to absorb UV light, terpenoids to attract pollinators or repel pests. Humans discovered these effects and repurposed them for medicine, exploiting nature's solutions to problems we share, such as infection, inflammation, or neurological imbalance. In other words, the medicinal efficacy of plants is a side effect of their survival strategy, an example of convergent utility across kingdoms.

Extraction and isolation, however, are only the beginning. Structural elucidation is where chemistry meets imagination. Consider paclitaxel (Taxol), a complex diterpenoid first extracted from the Pacific yew. Its intricate ring system (Figure 20) and oxygenation pattern were deciphered only through painstaking analysis, revealing not just a molecule but a blueprint of biological potential. This molecule, evolved to defend the tree against herbivores, now stabilizes microtubules in human cancer cells, halting cell division. Such stories illustrate the dual authorship of natural products: evolution and human curiosity collaborating across millennia.

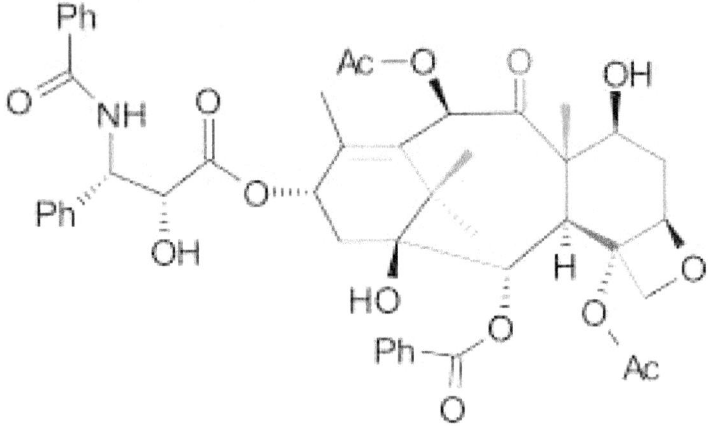

Figure 20. Paclitaxel. Dissolution, CC BY-SA 3.0 <https://creativecommons.org/licenses/by-sa/3.0>, via Wikimedia Commons

Biosynthetic pathways provide further insight and opportunity. Understanding how a plant or microbe assembles a molecule enables semi-synthetic or total synthesis, increasing yield, modifying activity, or producing analogs with improved pharmacokinetics. Artemisinin, the antimalarial sesquiterpene, was originally limited by the slow growth of *Artemisia annua* (Figure 21). Knowledge of its biosynthesis allowed researchers to engineer yeast to produce the compound efficiently, translating natural ingenuity into industrial feasibility. This interplay of observation, chemistry, and biotechnology is the hallmark of modern pharmacognosy.

History is rich with examples of this evolution from folk remedy to therapeutic mainstay. Vincristine and vinblastine, alkaloids from *Catharanthus roseus*, were discovered through ethnobotanical leads in Madagascar. These compounds, initially used in traditional medicine for diabetes, were found to inhibit microtubule formation, becoming cornerstone treatments for leukemia and lymphoma. Such discoveries highlight the layered narrative: evolution produces a molecule for defense, humans find an effect on physiology, and chemistry and biology convert it into a drug. Each step adds a chapter to the story.

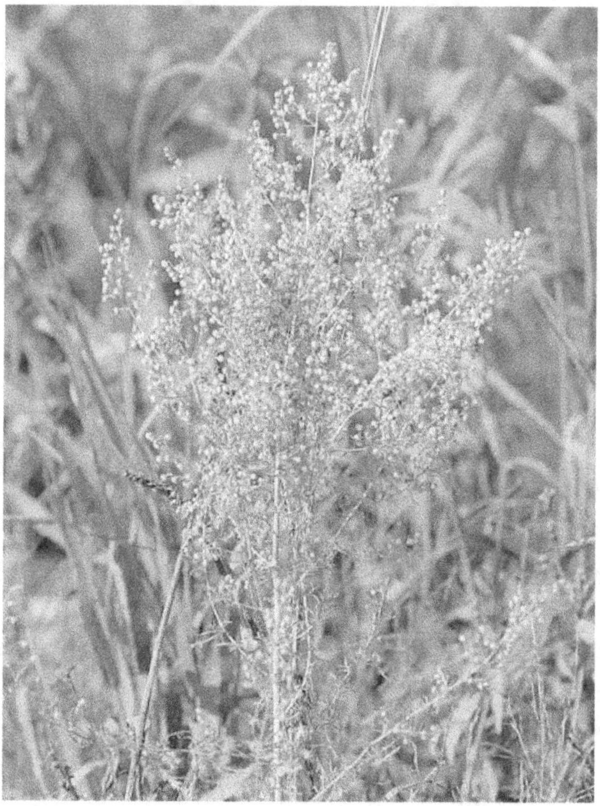

Figure 21. Artemisia annua. Kristian Peters -- Fabelfroh 11:39, 16 September 2007 (UTC), CC BY-SA 3.0 <http://creativecommons.org/licenses/by-sa/3.0/>, via Wikimedia Commons

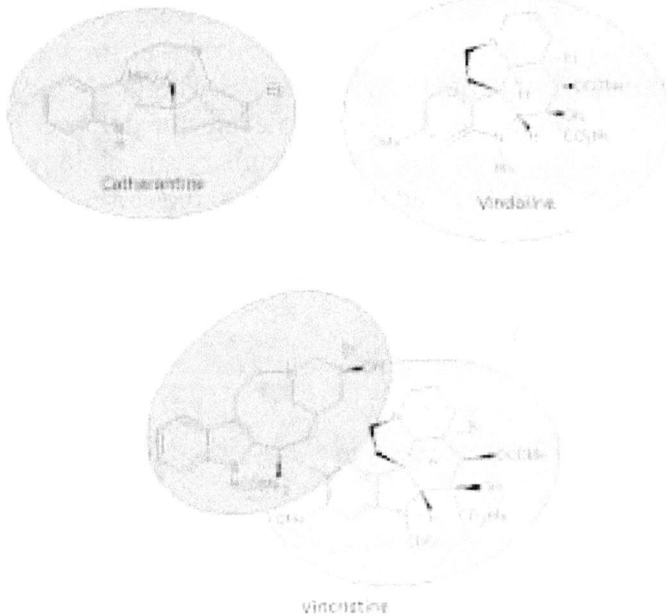

Figure 22. Vinca alkaloids derived from the Madagascar periwinkle. ClaraM-L2SVG, CC BY-SA 4.0 <https://creativecommons.org/licenses/by-sa/4.0>, via Wikimedia Commons

The narrative of discovery is also intertwined with ecological and cultural contexts. Plants, their metabolites, and the traditional knowledge surrounding them are products of specific habitats and communities. Protecting biodiversity is not only a moral imperative but a practical one: many potentially life-saving compounds remain hidden in threatened ecosystems, while their associated ethnobotanical wisdom is at risk of being lost. Intellectual property, benefit-sharing, and respect for indigenous knowledge are therefore critical elements in the modern story of pharmacognosy.

In practical terms, the transformation from traditional use to modern drug involves iterative validation. Bioactivity-guided fractionation screens compounds for desired effects. Toxicological studies ensure safety. Mechanistic studies uncover molecular targets, signaling pathways, and pharmacodynamics. The journey from a plant in the forest to a pill in a pharmacy is long, rigorous, and expensive. But it begins with the simple act of noticing which leaf heals and which does not. It is a testament to the interplay of observation, intuition, and scientific rigor.

Perhaps most compelling is the narrative continuity across millennia. The molecules humans exploit today (*e.g.,* quinine, morphine, taxol, artemisinin) are products of evolutionary strategies developed long before human arrival. Yet these strategies, when interpreted and adapted, become tools for human health. Modern pharmacognosy, therefore, is not the invention of new solutions but the intelligent reading of an ancient library of chemical innovation. Each molecule is a story: of survival, adaptation, and the serendipitous alignment of natural design with human need.

Finally, this chapter underscores the philosophy inherent in pharmacognosy: humans are participants, not creators. We read nature's chemical scripts, interpret their meanings, and apply them in ways that enhance our survival and well-being. In doing so, we become collaborators with evolutionary history, translators of biochemical language, and narrators of the ongoing story of life's ingenuity. The leaves, roots, and bark that once served as remedies for fevers, pain, or infection now occupy the shelves of modern medicine. Not because humans invented them, but because we learned to read, respect, and build upon the molecular narratives nature had already written.

CHAPTER 9: BIOSYNTHESIS GUIDES DRUG DISCOVERY

Nature has long been its own laboratory, assembling complex molecules with a precision and purpose that human chemists can only aspire to replicate. For millions of years, plants, fungi, and bacteria have been perfecting chemical defenses (*e.g.*, alkaloids to deter herbivores, terpenoids to repel predators, phenolics to ward off pathogens). These molecules, forged under selective pressures and ecological negotiation, became the hidden treasures that humans would eventually co-opt for medicine. Understanding the biosynthesis of these compounds (the pathways, enzymes, and structural logic) is the gateway to transforming natural products into therapeutic agents.

Take paclitaxel, known popularly as Taxol, as a striking example. When the bark of the Pacific yew, *Taxus brevifolia*, first revealed its anticancer potential, it astonished researchers not only because of its potency but because of the molecule's astonishing structural complexity: an eight-membered taxane ring system adorned with multiple oxygenated functional groups. Deciphering the biosynthetic pathway was no trivial task. Scientists traced the carbon skeleton back to the mevalonate pathway, which produces isopentenyl pyrophosphate (IPP), a five-carbon unit used in countless terpenoid structures. Through a cascade of enzymatic transformations—cyclization, hydroxylation, acetylation, and oxetane ring formation—nature built a molecule capable of stabilizing microtubules in cancer cells, arresting mitosis, and triggering apoptosis. Each enzymatic step was optimized by evolution, a testament to millions of years of chemical trial and error in the tree's survival strategy.

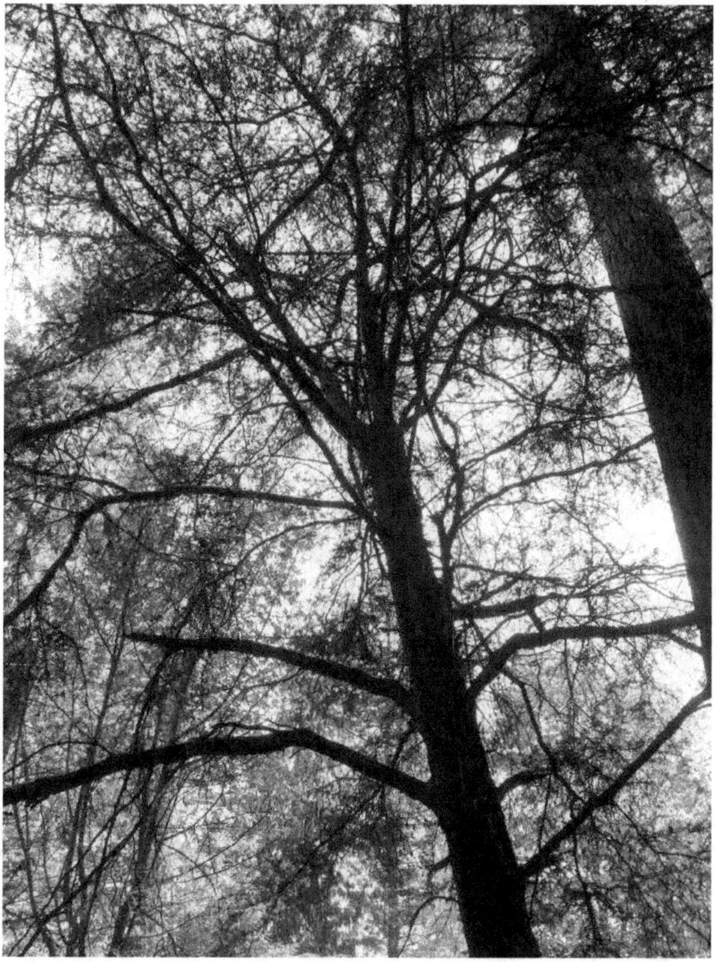

Figure 23. The Pacific Yew (Taxus breviflоia). brewbooks from near Seattle, USA, CC BY-SA 2.0 <https://creativecommons.org/licenses/by-sa/2.0>, via Wikimedia Commons

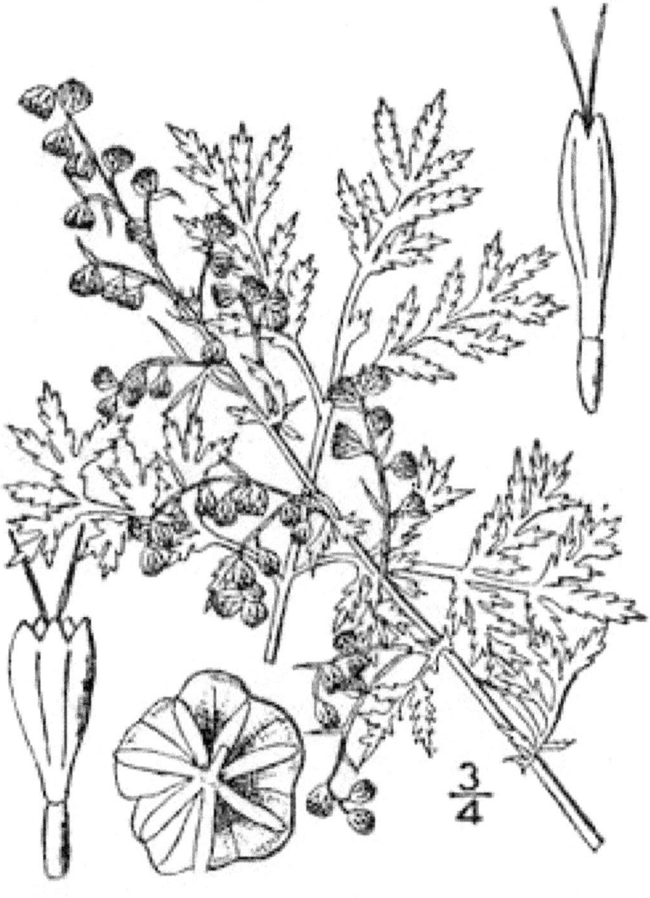

Figure 24. Sweet wormwood. USDA-NRCS PLANTS Database / Britton, N.L., and A. Brown. 1913. Illustrated flora of the northern states and Canada. Vol. 3: 526.

The human journey to harness paclitaxel was equally complex. Initial extraction from yew bark was ecologically unsustainable, threatening the species and requiring tons of bark for mere grams of the drug. Semi-synthetic approaches using precursors from renewable sources, coupled with biotechnological production in cell cultures, eventually solved this problem. Researchers could now replicate, and even modify, nature's construction with remarkable fidelity, demonstrating that understanding the biosynthetic logic of a molecule enables human ingenuity to collaborate with evolutionary intelligence.

Artemisinin, the antimalarial compound derived from *Artemisia annua*, tells a similar story. Folk healers in China had long used sweet wormwood tea for fever, a practice dismissed by Western science for centuries. It was only through systematic investigation that artemisinin was isolated and its molecular basis elucidated. Biosynthetically, artemisinin arises from the mevalonate pathway, producing farnesyl pyrophosphate (FPP), which is cyclized into amorpha-4,11-diene and subsequently oxygenated to yield the endoperoxide pharmacophore essential for antimalarial activity. The discovery of its pathway did more than explain nature's logic; it enabled microbial engineering, producing artemisinin precursors in yeast at industrial scale. This bridging of evolution, ethnobotany, and biotechnology exemplifies how biosynthetic insight translates into human utility.

The Madagascar periwinkle, *Catharanthus roseus*, offers yet another remarkable case. Its alkaloids vincristine and vinblastine, now cornerstones in cancer chemotherapy, arise from the indole alkaloid biosynthetic pathway. Beginning with tryptophan, the plant assembles strictosidine (a central intermediate) from which an astonishing diversity of bioactive molecules emerges. The pathway is intricate: multiple methylations, oxidations, and glycosylations converge to produce compounds that disrupt microtubule formation in malignant cells. Early researchers faced immense challenges, isolating these molecules in minute quantities from delicate plant tissues. Only through careful mapping of the biosynthetic pathway and eventual microbial and plant cell engineering did production become scalable.

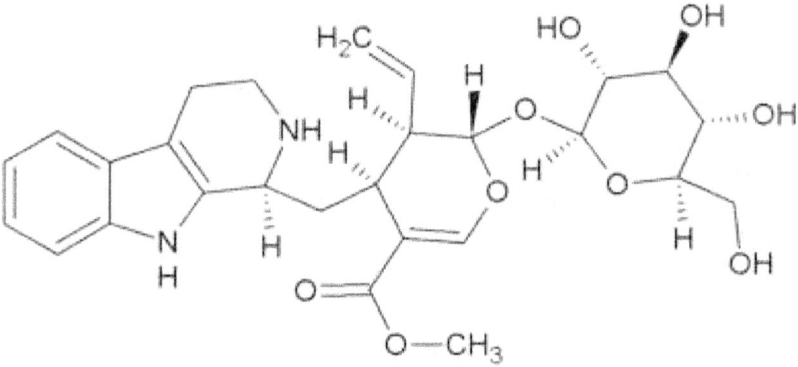

Figure 25. Strictosidine. Cmsc236, CC BY-SA 4.0 <https://creativecommons.org/licenses/by-sa/4.0>, via Wikimedia Commons

What these examples share is a common theme: biosynthetic pathways are evolutionary strategies writ in chemical form. Plants and microbes did not evolve these molecules to serve human medicine; they evolved them to survive, compete, and communicate. Yet humans, by decoding these pathways, gain access to a treasure trove of chemical ingenuity. Each enzyme, each precursor, each cyclization or oxidation step is a lesson in evolutionary design, revealing how nature solves complex chemical problems.

The study of biosynthesis also illuminates co-evolution and symbiosis. Endophytic fungi, for instance, may contribute key enzymes or intermediates in plant secondary metabolite pathways. The discovery of *Taxomyces andreanae*, an endophytic fungus producing paclitaxel, underscores the hidden collaborative dimension: the plant and its microbial partners jointly construct molecules with sophisticated structures and bioactivity. Horizontal gene transfer among microbes further accelerates chemical innovation, allowing pathways to be reshuffled, modified, or combined in novel ways. Understanding these networks is critical not only for appreciating evolution but for designing strategies to enhance drug production.

Modern drug discovery increasingly leverages this knowledge. Combinatorial biosynthesis, for example, involves swapping, duplicating, or mutating enzymatic modules within biosynthetic pathways to create new molecules that nature has not yet evolved. By manipulating polyketide synthases or nonribosomal peptide synthetases, scientists generate structural diversity that can be screened for improved therapeutic properties—higher potency, reduced toxicity, or better pharmacokinetics. Such innovation relies on an intimate understanding of enzyme specificity, substrate flexibility, and pathway regulation, all learned from careful study of natural biosynthesis.

Synthetic biology adds yet another layer of sophistication. With gene editing and high-throughput sequencing, entire biosynthetic pathways can be reconstructed in microbial hosts. E. coli, yeast, and filamentous fungi can now serve as "factory floors," producing complex natural products without relying on slow-growing or rare plants. This approach not only conserves biodiversity but allows precise modification of chemical structures, optimizing drugs for human use. The process often involves iterative cycles: modeling enzyme kinetics, redesigning pathway modules, and testing outputs. It is a modern echo of the iterative, selective pressures that shaped the pathways in nature.

The biosynthetic story also carries lessons about human intuition and observation. Many drug discoveries start with a molecule known in folk medicine, whose active principle and biosynthesis are later elucidated. The integration of ethnobotanical knowledge, chemical analysis, and molecular biology exemplifies a continuum of learning, from observation, to chemical understanding, to engineering. It is a narrative in which humans become interpreters of evolutionary intelligence, rather than sole creators.

Finally, the ecological and ethical dimensions must be considered. Harvesting plants for bioactive compounds can threaten ecosystems if done unsustainably. Conservation, combined with microbial or plant cell engineering, preserves biodiversity while maintaining access to medicinal molecules. Recognizing the collaborative network of plants, microbes, and humans reframes pharmacognosy as not merely chemistry, but stewardship: guiding nature's creativity toward human benefit without diminishing its ecological foundation.

In sum, biosynthesis is the bridge between natural product chemistry and modern medicine. Understanding how evolution assembles molecules provides insight into their functions, guides drug discovery, and enables human engineering of new therapeutics. From paclitaxel stabilizing cancer microtubules to artemisinin quenching malaria parasites, the molecules we harness are evolutionary triumphs, and the pathways that produce them are blueprints of life's ingenuity. By studying and manipulating these pathways, we continue the collaboration with nature, translating millennia of chemical innovation into tools for human health, while remaining ever mindful of the ecological and evolutionary context from which they arose.

CHAPTER 10: STORIES OF LANDMARK DRUGS

Few stories in science are as compelling as those of discovery, serendipity, and the slow unravelling of nature's secrets. In pharmacognosy, these stories are written in molecules: quinine, morphine, paclitaxel, artemisinin, vincristine. These are compounds that began as plants' defenses against herbivores, microbes, and environmental stress, and ended as cornerstones of human medicine. Each drug tells a narrative not just of chemistry, but of observation, trial, and human perseverance intertwined with evolutionary history.

Consider quinine, the first antimalarial to capture global attention. For centuries, indigenous peoples of the Andean forests knew that the bark of *Cinchona* trees could reduce fever. European colonists, arriving in South America, observed this remedy and began systematic extraction, translating centuries of empirical knowledge into a laboratory context. Chemists eventually isolated quinine, a bitter alkaloid with a remarkable ability to disrupt the life cycle of *Plasmodium* parasites. Its biosynthesis, originating from the shikimate pathway leading to complex aromatic structures, illustrates evolution's ingenuity: a molecule shaped to deter herbivores also interferes with a unicellular eukaryotic parasite. The story of quinine is also a tale of geopolitics, colonialism, and the race to secure medicinal resources, reminding us that human history is inseparable from natural products discovery.

Morphine offers another vivid narrative. The latex of *Papaver somniferum*, the opium poppy, has been used for millennia as an analgesic and sedative. Ancient civilizations documented its effects in texts and artifacts, yet the molecule itself remained hidden within the latex. In the early 19th century, Friedrich Sertürner (Figure 27) isolated morphine, transforming a crude extract into a chemically defined compound. Its biosynthesis, a cascade from tyrosine through dopamine-like intermediates to complex benzylisoquinoline structures, represents a sophisticated defensive strategy of the plant. Morphine deters herbivores, yet humans discovered its analgesic power, highlighting the serendipitous overlap of evolutionary and therapeutic utility. The story continues today with semi-synthetic derivatives, illustrating how knowledge of biosynthesis guides modern drug development.

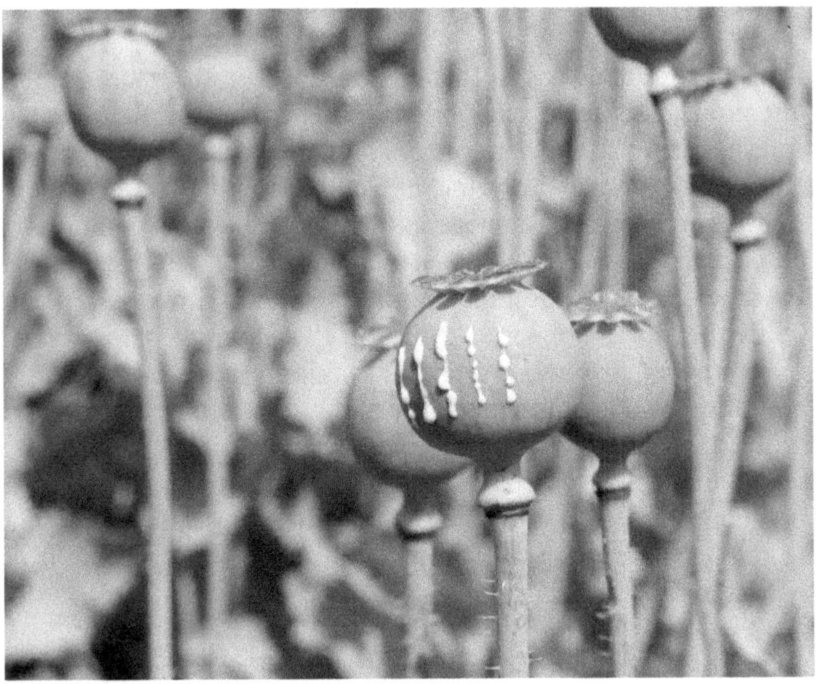

Figure 26. Opium poppy (Papaver somniferum). George Chernilevsky, CC BY-SA 4.0 <https://creativecommons.org/licenses/by-sa/4.0>, via Wikimedia Commons

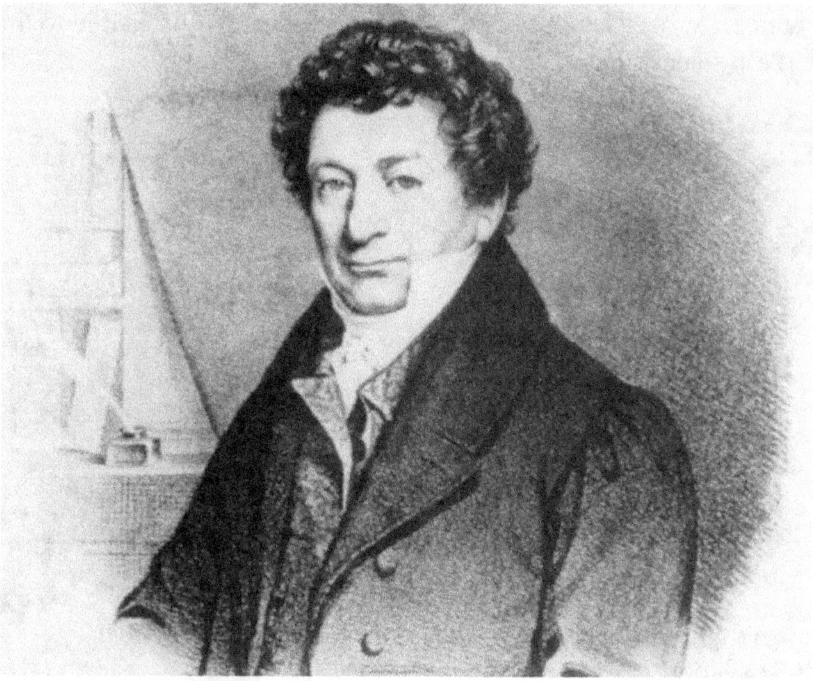

Figure 27. Lithography of the German pharmacist Friedrich Sertürner. He discovered morphine in 1804. Julius Giere, Public domain, via Wikimedia Commons

Paclitaxel, as introduced in the previous chapter, combines botanical rarity with molecular sophistication. Extracted from the bark of the Pacific yew, it stabilizes microtubules in cancer cells, arresting division and inducing apoptosis. Its discovery exemplifies the convergence of ethnobotany, natural product chemistry, and evolutionary insight. Unlike morphine or quinine, paclitaxel was not initially used in folk medicine; its activity was uncovered through systematic screening of thousands of plant extracts. Here, the evolutionary narrative is silent yet profound: the tree evolved a complex diterpenoid as a chemical defense, which humans later repurposed to combat cancer, a disease that, in evolutionary terms, was invisible to the tree's selective pressures.

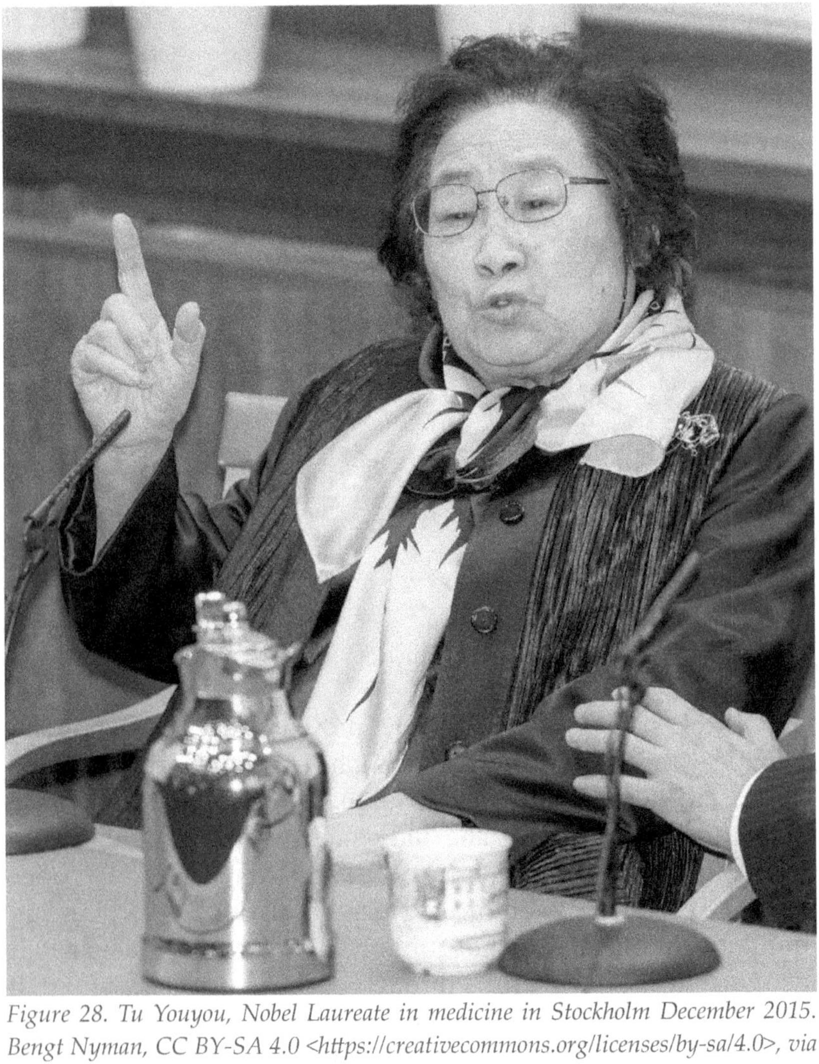

Figure 28. Tu Youyou, Nobel Laureate in medicine in Stockholm December 2015. Bengt Nyman, CC BY-SA 4.0 <https://creativecommons.org/licenses/by-sa/4.0>, via Wikimedia Commons

Artemisinin, the antimalarial compound, bridges folk knowledge and modern science in a particularly elegant way. Chinese healers had long known that tea made from *Artemisia annua* reduced fevers, yet the active component remained elusive. In the 1970s, under a secret project during a national health crisis, Tu Youyou isolated artemisinin, characterized its structure, and demonstrated its remarkable efficacy against malaria. Its biosynthesis, a series of oxidations of amorpha-4,11-diene, underscores the intricate enzymatic orchestration of natural molecules. The story of artemisinin illustrates a recurrent theme in pharmacognosy: evolution crafts molecules for ecological survival, humans discover their utility through observation and analysis, and technology enables scalable application.

Vincristine and vinblastine, alkaloids from *Catharanthus roseus*, further exemplify the intersection of evolution, chemistry, and medicine. Indigenous populations in Madagascar used the plant traditionally, but its anticancer potential emerged only in the mid-20th century. The compounds inhibit microtubule assembly, halting the proliferation of malignant cells. Their complex indole alkaloid structures arise from intricate pathways beginning with tryptophan, demonstrating nature's combinatorial creativity. Efforts to isolate these compounds in sufficient quantity challenged chemists for decades, prompting innovations in cell culture, semi-synthesis, and eventually microbial production.

Across these stories, one pattern emerges: humans are interpreters of evolutionary narratives. The molecules discovered were not designed for human use, yet their effects resonate with our physiology. Evolution, driven by selection pressures on plants and microbes, generates chemical diversity and specificity; humans, through observation, isolation, and synthesis, recognize and harness this diversity for health. Biosynthetic pathways reveal the logic behind these molecules, guiding chemists to replicate, modify, and scale production.

These landmark drugs also illustrate the iterative nature of discovery. Early successes often depended on serendipity: observing the effects of bark, latex, or leaf extracts. Subsequent research required rigorous chemical analysis, structural elucidation, and pharmacological testing. Each step built upon the last, layering knowledge from ethnobotany, biochemistry, molecular biology, and clinical science. Evolution provided the molecular blueprint, and human ingenuity deciphered it.

Another common thread is sustainability and conservation. Paclitaxel's initial extraction threatened the Pacific yew, highlighting the need to balance discovery with ecological stewardship. Artemisinin's production initially relied on slow-growing *Artemisia* plants, prompting biotechnological innovations in yeast and other microbial systems. In each case, understanding biosynthesis allowed humans to respect ecological limits while still harnessing the molecule's potential. This is a theme that underscores modern pharmacognosy's ethical dimension.

The narratives of these drugs are not only chemical or historical; they are stories of collaboration across time and species. Endophytic fungi, soil microbes, and plant metabolic networks all contribute to the molecules' existence. Humans enter as both observers and engineers, guided by curiosity and empathy for life. Each compound is a testament to the coalescence of evolutionary strategy, chemical creativity, and human discovery.

Further, these landmark drugs offer lessons for the future. New challenges (*i.e.,* antibiotic resistance, emerging infectious diseases, cancer) demand molecules as sophisticated and multifaceted as those we have inherited from nature. By studying past successes, including the evolutionary origins, biosynthetic pathways, and human ingenuity involved, pharmacognosists can anticipate new compounds, design innovative screening methods, and engineer microbes or plants to produce them efficiently. The stories of quinine, morphine, paclitaxel, artemisinin, and vincristine thus become templates, guiding contemporary drug discovery.

Ultimately, the tale of landmark drugs is a narrative of connectivity: between plants, microbes, and humans; between evolution and medicine; between chemistry and ecology. Each molecule carries with it a legacy of adaptation and survival, now translated into human health benefits. The stories remind us that pharmacognosy is more than a catalog of molecules; it is the study of relationships, of dialogue across species and time, of intelligence embedded in matter, waiting to be interpreted.

Walking through a forest, one might see only leaves, bark, and flowers. Yet within each organism, a library of chemical innovation awaits, each molecule a story of survival, each pathway a record of evolutionary ingenuity. The human task is to read these stories, to understand their context, and to apply them responsibly, translating millions of years of natural experimentation into life-saving medicine. Landmark drugs are milestones on this journey—proof that by listening carefully to nature, humans can discover remedies, insights, and inspiration far beyond what we could invent on our own.

PART IV

DUKAS: OPEN PATHWAYS FOR THE FUTURE

CHAPTER 11: SYNTHETIC BIOLOGY AND DESIGNER MOLECULES

In the quiet hum of a modern laboratory, something extraordinary occurs: scientists coax microbes into becoming chemists, weaving molecules that no plant or fungus had yet imagined. Synthetic biology is a frontier where evolution's ancient logic meets human creativity, a place where the molecular narratives of life are read, interpreted, and rewritten. Just as our ancestors observed leaves, bark, and flowers for clues to their medicinal potential, today's researchers peer into genomes, enzyme structures, and metabolic networks, seeking to understand nature's chemical grammar, and to improvise upon it.

At the heart of this enterprise lies a profound realization: the molecules that plants, fungi, and bacteria produce are not random. Every terpenoid, alkaloid, flavonoid, and polyketide is the product of millions of years of evolutionary trial and error. These compounds are solutions to ecological problems (*i.e.*, defending tissues, attracting pollinators, deterring herbivores, or communicating with symbionts). By decoding the biosynthetic pathways that generate these molecules, scientists acquire more than a map of chemical reactions; they gain insight into the principles of molecular construction, modularity, and functional diversity.

Consider the story of artemisinin once more. Its discovery, rooted in folk knowledge and classical extraction techniques, eventually led to microbial engineering. Researchers transferred genes from *Artemisia annua* into yeast, enabling the fermentation of artemisinic acid, a precursor of artemisinin. This transformation, from plant to microbial factory, was more than a technological feat. It was a narrative of collaboration across species, time, and knowledge traditions. Evolution had designed the molecule for ecological survival, humans discovered its utility against malaria, and synthetic biology allowed its scalable production, preserving both the plant and human lives.

Synthetic biology builds upon such examples, but it also ventures beyond them. By understanding the modular logic of enzymes (how one catalytic domain adds a methyl group, another oxidizes a carbon, and yet another cyclizes a chain) researchers can rearrange these modules to generate "designer molecules." Polyketide synthases and nonribosomal peptide synthetases, the molecular assembly lines of natural products, can be recombined, truncated, or mutated to produce chemical scaffolds never observed in nature. In essence, humans are becoming co-authors in evolution's molecular narrative, blending the old stories with novel possibilities.

The implications of this work are profound. Imagine a cancer therapy molecule whose structure is informed by paclitaxel but engineered for improved solubility and reduced side effects, or an antibiotic inspired by erythromycin yet designed to overcome resistance mechanisms. Each of these compounds is a testament to a multilayered dialogue: the plant evolved the original molecule, scientists deciphered its biosynthesis, and synthetic biology allows us to iterate on it with precision. The story is evolutionary, chemical, and human simultaneously.

Yet this endeavor is not merely technical; it is philosophical. To manipulate life's molecular machinery is to engage with evolution in a deliberate and conscious way. Each gene inserted into a microbial host, each pathway optimized, is a negotiation with natural laws. The enzymes, evolved over eons to operate in specific contexts, must be coaxed to function in new environments. The microbes, small and silent collaborators, respond in unpredictable ways, sometimes producing unexpected side products that open new avenues of discovery. Science becomes a conversation with evolution itself, a collaboration where humans and microbes co-create solutions.

The history of designer molecules is punctuated by both triumph and humility. Early attempts at pathway reconstruction often failed, revealing the subtlety of enzyme interactions and the necessity of cellular context. For instance, attempts to produce taxol analogs in bacteria initially stumbled because the host lacked the proper subcellular compartments to support enzyme activity. Only through careful redesign of enzyme localization, cofactor provision, and pathway balancing could productive synthesis occur. Each challenge revealed hidden lessons: the importance of spatial organization, metabolic flux, and regulatory networks, echoing the complexity that evolution had encoded in the plant.

Beyond single compounds, synthetic biology allows the creation of entire libraries of molecules, each a small variation on a theme. By systematically altering enzyme specificity, substrate availability, or pathway topology, researchers generate chemical diversity that rivals, and sometimes exceeds, natural variation. These libraries become playgrounds for discovery: each molecule is screened for biological activity, potential toxicity, or pharmacokinetic advantage. In this sense, evolution's principle of variation and selection is mirrored in the laboratory, but accelerated by human ingenuity and high-throughput technologies.

Synthetic biology also intersects with ecology and conservation. By producing rare or endangered plant metabolites in microbial hosts, we relieve pressure on natural populations while preserving access to life-saving compounds. This approach reflects a growing ethos in pharmacognosy: discovery and innovation must coexist with stewardship. Just as indigenous knowledge preserved centuries of empirical observation, modern science can honor and protect the ecosystems that inspired these molecules, translating respect for biodiversity into sustainable pharmaceutical practice.

The philosophical resonance of this work is compelling. Humans are not merely extractors of nature's wealth; we are interpreters, collaborators, and storytellers. Each designer molecule is a narrative co-authored with evolution: the enzyme that catalyzes a cyclization, the microbe that hosts the pathway, the researcher who optimizes production, they all contribute to a story that spans kingdoms and millennia. In this way, synthetic biology does not replace nature's ingenuity. It amplifies it, extending the molecular dialogue into realms that evolution alone may never have explored.

The field is rapidly expanding. CRISPR-mediated gene editing, high-throughput screening, computational pathway modeling, and machine learning-guided enzyme design are enabling feats unimaginable even a decade ago. A molecule inspired by a plant defense can now be rationally modified for improved activity, produced in a microbial host at industrial scale, and screened against dozens of disease models in parallel. The laboratory has become both observatory and workshop, reading evolution's chemical scripts and composing new chapters.

Ultimately, synthetic biology is a continuation of the story that began with human curiosity in the forests, the mountains, and the fields. Just as our ancestors observed which leaves soothed pain or reduced fever, today's scientists observe, decode, and innovate on nature's molecular inventions. Designer molecules are the product of a multilayered narrative: evolution provides the original script, humans interpret and extend it, and the laboratory becomes a stage where molecules perform roles neither plant nor herbivore could have anticipated.

As we peer into this future, one truth becomes clear: the molecules themselves are storytellers. Paclitaxel tells of a tree defending against herbivory. Artemisinin speaks of a plant and its ecosystem, discovered by observant healers. Vincristine narrates an intricate chemical ballet orchestrated over millennia. Synthetic biology allows us to read these stories in full, understand the underlying grammar, and even craft new narratives, writing molecules that address challenges humanity has never faced before.

In the end, the discipline is more than chemistry or biology; it is a philosophy of engagement with life's ingenuity. Each pathway elucidated, each enzyme harnessed, each designer molecule produced is a testament to the continuity between evolution, observation, and innovation. Through synthetic biology, we do not conquer nature. Instead, we converse with it, translating millions of years of molecular adaptation into therapeutic solutions for a modern world.

CHAPTER 12: CONSERVATION AND ETHICS

In the depths of tropical forests, among moss-draped trees and whispering streams, lie the secrets of countless molecules, each a product of survival, adaptation, and intricate ecological negotiation. These molecules (*e.g.*, alkaloids, terpenoids, polyketides) are the silent witnesses to a drama millions of years in the making. For centuries, humans have benefitted from them, translating bark, leaves, and roots into remedies and medicines. Yet with this access comes responsibility. Conservation and ethics are no longer optional footnotes in pharmacognosy; they are essential chapters, without which the story of drug discovery is incomplete.

The narrative of conservation begins with recognition: the plants, fungi, and microbes that provide medicinal compounds are finite, fragile, and often under threat. The Pacific yew, whose bark once yielded paclitaxel, is a prime example. Early extraction methods demanded harvesting vast quantities of slow-growing trees, threatening local populations and ecosystems. Without intervention, humanity risked depleting not just a resource, but a living archive of chemical innovation. Similarly, rare species of *Artemisia*, the source of artemisinin, grow in limited regions with fragile ecological balances. Here, the chemical narratives that evolution painstakingly wrote were intertwined with environmental stability; their survival depended on maintaining habitats, soil integrity, and symbiotic microbial partners.

Ethical considerations extend beyond ecology. Traditional knowledge accumulated over generations by indigenous peoples and local healers often provides the first clues to bioactive compounds. Willow bark, *Cinchona*, and *Catharanthus roseus* carry stories preserved in cultural memory. The challenge arises when pharmaceutical development extracts molecules or knowledge without proper recognition or benefit-sharing. History is littered with examples of knowledge appropriated, communities marginalized, and resources exploited. Ethical pharmacognosy requires acknowledgment: crediting traditional knowledge holders, negotiating equitable benefits, and protecting intellectual property in ways that respect cultural context.

The story of artemisinin illustrates the intertwining of ethics, conservation, and discovery. Tu Youyou's work drew on centuries of Chinese herbal medicine. Yet the broader deployment of artemisinin also highlighted global inequalities in access to medicine, intellectual property disputes, and the ethics of commercialization. Preserving the ecological source (*i.e.,* the *Artemisia annua* plants) was as vital as ensuring fair distribution of the drug. Here, ethical stewardship became inseparable from scientific success.

Conservation in pharmacognosy is not a passive act of avoidance but a creative challenge. Scientists have developed strategies to reduce ecological pressure while sustaining innovation. Microbial fermentation, plant cell cultures, and synthetic biology allow production of valuable molecules without harvesting wild populations. For example, microbial production of paclitaxel precursors reduces demand on yew trees, while yeast-based artemisinin production preserves *Artemisia* populations. Each technical advance is, in effect, a story of human collaboration with nature: evolution designed the molecule, humans read its instructions, and technology allows production in ways that respect ecological limits.

Yet conservation also demands attention to less visible elements of ecosystems. Secondary metabolites often depend on symbiotic interactions. Endophytic fungi, nitrogen-fixing bacteria, and soil microbiomes contribute to the plant's ability to synthesize complex molecules. Disrupting these relationships (*e.g.*, through deforestation, monoculture, or chemical pollution) can collapse biosynthetic potential. Preserving chemical diversity therefore entails preserving ecological networks, not merely individual species. The narrative of pharmacognosy is inseparable from the narrative of life itself, in all its interconnected complexity.

Ethics extends to human engagement with these natural networks. Modern pharmacognosy sits at a junction: scientists hold the power to translate chemical diversity into therapeutics, yet with this power comes moral responsibility. Equitable benefit-sharing, recognition of indigenous contributions, and legal frameworks that prevent exploitation are not bureaucratic hurdles; they are part of the story, ensuring that knowledge, wealth, and opportunity are fairly distributed. Without these considerations, discovery risks becoming a tale of extraction and inequity, undermining the humanistic aspect that underpins the field.

Education plays a crucial role in this ethical framework. By teaching new generations of scientists to appreciate the stories embedded in molecules, pharmacognosy instills a sense of stewardship alongside discovery. Students learn that each molecule represents an ecosystem, a lineage, and a cultural narrative. They learn that laboratories are not isolated arenas of production but extensions of natural and social networks. Ethics, in this sense, is inseparable from science; it is embedded in the very act of observation, extraction, and innovation.

Consider a rainforest where a rare alkaloid is discovered. The ethical scientist does not simply harvest and patent. They observe the plant's ecological role, understand its interactions with pollinators and microbes, engage with local communities who have long valued it, and design sustainable methods of production. Microbial engineering, plant cell culture, and pathway elucidation become not just technical solutions but ethical strategies, harmonizing human needs with ecological and cultural preservation. Each molecule thus carries layers of meaning: evolutionary adaptation, human ingenuity, ecological context, and ethical responsibility.

Global collaboration amplifies this responsibility. As pharmacognosy becomes increasingly international, harmonizing ethical standards is vital. Sharing genomic data, biosynthetic pathways, and chemical libraries across borders must be balanced with respect for local sovereignty, biodiversity regulations, and benefit-sharing frameworks. Open science and equitable collaboration can accelerate discovery while maintaining ethical integrity, ensuring that the story of pharmacognosy remains one of respect, cooperation, and shared curiosity.

Conservation and ethics are, ultimately, part of a larger narrative: the ongoing story of life's chemical ingenuity and humanity's engagement with it. Evolution writes the molecules; humans discover, interpret, and engineer them; and ethical principles guide the way these discoveries are applied and shared. Without consideration of these dimensions, pharmacognosy risks becoming a tale of shortsighted exploitation, disconnected from the ecological and cultural networks that sustain both molecules and people.

The beauty of this narrative lies in its continuity. From the first herbalist observing the soothing effects of a leaf, to chemists deciphering complex structures, to synthetic biologists engineering new pathways, each step is connected by curiosity, respect, and responsibility. Conservation and ethics are not interruptions to this story; they are integral chapters, ensuring that the dialogue between humans and nature remains rich, sustainable, and just.

As we look forward, the stakes grow ever higher. Emerging diseases, antibiotic resistance, and the ongoing loss of biodiversity demand that pharmacognosy remains vigilant, adaptive, and principled. The molecules we discover today (guided by evolution, informed by tradition, and optimized by science) must be harvested, produced, and shared in ways that honor the ecosystems and communities from which they originate. Every leaf, root, fungus, or microbe carries a narrative that extends beyond chemistry; it embodies relationships, history, and ethical obligations. To ignore these is to silence part of the story, to sever a link in the chain that connects life, knowledge, and human health.

In the end, conservation and ethics are not separate from discovery; they are discovery's most profound extension. They remind us that pharmacognosy is a story of collaboration across time, species, and cultures. Each molecule is a testament to evolution, each pathway a record of survival, each innovation a negotiation between human curiosity and natural wisdom. By preserving biodiversity, honoring traditional knowledge, and applying ethical stewardship, we ensure that the story continues—an unbroken narrative of life's chemical genius, interpreted and respected by those who seek to learn, heal, and create.

CONCLUSION: THE ONGOING STORY

If pharmacognosy has taught us anything, it is that life is a storyteller, and molecules are its language. From the shadowed floors of tropical forests to the high-tech fermenters of modern laboratories, nature has been composing narratives in chemistry, encoding survival strategies, ecological dialogues, and evolutionary experiments in terpenoids, alkaloids, polyketides, and flavonoids. Each compound carries a history: a lineage of adaptation, a tale of chemical ingenuity, and a story of interaction with the world. Humans have long been eavesdroppers in this narrative, first by observation, then by extraction, and now by collaboration and innovation.

The journey begins with curiosity. Ancient healers observed leaves that soothed pain, bark that reduced fevers, and roots that eased inflammation. Their observations were careful, empirical, and grounded in lived experience. Quinine, morphine, vincristine, and artemisinin were hidden within these practices, awaiting the lens of chemistry to reveal their molecular structure and pharmacological potential. Evolution, operating over millions of years, had already solved complex chemical problems, selecting for molecules that were biologically active, stereochemically precise, and ecologically functional. Humans discovered not the molecules themselves (they had been there all along) but the principles underlying their creation.

Biosynthetic pathways are the bridge between evolutionary design and human application. They explain how plants and microbes assemble molecules with precision, orchestrating enzymes and precursors to yield compounds that are at once complex and purposeful. Paclitaxel's taxane ring, artemisinin's endoperoxide bridge, vincristine's indole alkaloid scaffold, all are chemical architectures that evolution engineered as defenses, yet humans repurposed them for healing. Understanding these pathways is not merely a scientific exercise; it is an act of interpretation, a translation of nature's language into human utility.

The story deepens when we consider the evolutionary logic behind these molecules. Plants do not create paclitaxel to treat cancer, nor artemisinin to combat malaria. Each molecule arises as a solution to ecological challenges: deterring herbivores, resisting pathogens, communicating with pollinators, or collaborating with microbial symbionts. By recognizing these evolutionary narratives, humans gain insight into the chemical diversity that surrounds them. Evolution teaches us that the same molecule may serve multiple functions, that minor modifications can alter activity profoundly, and that biological context matters. These are lessons that guide modern drug discovery.

Synthetic biology extends this narrative into a new realm. Where evolution provided the original blueprint, humans now act as co-authors, rearranging, optimizing, and designing molecules with precision. Microbes become chemical factories, enzymes are coaxed into new roles, and metabolic pathways are reconstructed to produce natural products sustainably. Yet even in this technological arena, the story remains collaborative: humans read and interpret evolution's chemical scripts, respecting their logic while introducing novelty. Paclitaxel analogs engineered for solubility, artemisinin produced in yeast at scale, combinatorial libraries of polyketides, all these demonstrate that discovery and creation are continuous dialogues between natural intelligence and human ingenuity.

Ethics and conservation form another chapter in this ongoing story. The molecules we seek are not isolated entities but products of ecological networks, symbioses, and cultural knowledge. Overharvesting threatens biodiversity; neglecting traditional knowledge risks exploitation and inequity. Ethical pharmacognosy demands that we recognize these relationships, designing sustainable production methods, honoring indigenous knowledge, and sharing benefits equitably. Conservation is thus inseparable from innovation: protecting habitats preserves not just species but chemical potential, ensuring that future generations can participate in the molecular dialogue.

Human stories are interwoven with these molecular and ecological narratives. Chemists who painstakingly isolated compounds, ethnobotanists who documented traditional practices, biotechnologists who engineered microbes, all contribute to a continuum of knowledge. Serendipity, patience, ingenuity, and empathy have been as essential as laboratory techniques. The story of Tu Youyou and artemisinin illustrates this beautifully: centuries of folk medicine informed rigorous scientific inquiry, culminating in a discovery that has saved millions of lives. Such examples remind us that science is as much a human endeavor as it is a chemical one.

The narrative also reveals the iterative nature of discovery. Molecules isolated centuries ago continue to inspire innovation, from semi-synthetic derivatives to fully engineered analogs. Lessons from quinine inform malaria treatment strategies, morphine guides analgesic drug design, paclitaxel inspires new anticancer scaffolds, and artemisinin directs modern synthetic biology approaches. Pharmacognosy is therefore a living story, where each discovery feeds the next, and evolution continues to provide templates and inspiration.

Conservation, ethics, and innovation are intertwined. Microbial production reduces pressure on endangered plants, metabolic engineering enables sustainable synthesis, and equitable frameworks ensure that traditional knowledge is respected. Each step reinforces the narrative that pharmacognosy is not merely the study of molecules, but the stewardship of life's chemical creativity. By preserving ecosystems, honoring cultures, and advancing technology, humans become responsible participants in the molecular dialogue, rather than exploiters of it.

As we contemplate the molecules themselves, one sees stories embedded in every bond, every functional group, every stereocenter. The taxane ring tells of a yew tree's struggle to survive herbivory, the endoperoxide bridge of artemisinin speaks to a plant's microbial environment, and vincristine's indole scaffold reflects a chemical dialogue shaped by evolution and ecological pressures. These molecules are time capsules, recording both the ancient past and the ongoing story of adaptation, survival, and chemical ingenuity.

Looking forward, the story continues. Emerging diseases, climate change, and biodiversity loss challenge humans to innovate responsibly. Synthetic biology, combinatorial chemistry, and microbial engineering offer powerful tools, but they must be guided by the principles learned from centuries of observation: respect for ecological networks, recognition of cultural knowledge, and understanding of evolutionary logic. Each molecule discovered or engineered is both a solution and a responsibility, a continuation of the dialogue that began in the forests, fields, and microbial mats of the natural world.

In the end, pharmacognosy is a story of connection: between species, across time, and between chemistry and culture.

Evolution writes the first draft; humans interpret, adapt, and innovate, always in conversation with the ecological and ethical context. Each drug, each pathway, each engineered molecule is a narrative thread, woven into a tapestry that spans millennia and continents. By reading, understanding, and respecting these stories, we become more than scientists or chemists; we become participants in the ongoing drama of life itself.

The molecules may be small, but their stories are vast. They remind us that discovery is not a solitary act but a dialogue, that chemical innovation is inseparable from ecological and cultural context, and that humans are both stewards and storytellers. The ongoing story of pharmacognosy is thus a narrative of wonder, responsibility, and collaboration: a testament to the ingenuity of life and the insight of those who seek to understand it.

As you close this book, remember: the next molecule you encounter, be it in a leaf, a microbe, or a laboratory, is more than chemistry. It is history, ecology, evolution, and human ingenuity intertwined. Its story is still unfolding, and in studying it, you become part of that narrative, a participant in the grand molecular drama that began long before us and will continue until the end of the world.

Sandiwâ Press is an independent publishing house dedicated to works that unite science, culture, and creativity. *Sandiwa*, from the Filipino words *isang diwa* ("one spirit"), embodies the vision of knowledge as a shared human endeavor. Its publications highlight scholarship, storytelling, and cultural depth, with a commitment to producing works that are both intellectually rigorous and accessible to a wider readership.

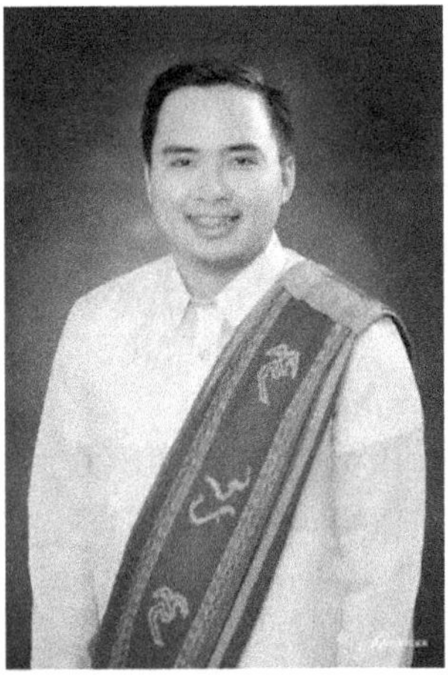

Brian Pollo is a physician-educator and writer whose works explore the intersections of medicine, science, and the humanities. His academic background in biochemistry, pharmacology, and clinical practice informs his teaching and research, while his passion for history, literature, and Filipino heritage shapes his creative writing. Through his books, he seeks to make complex knowledge accessible, weaving together scholarship, storytelling, and cultural imagination. His works are published under Sandiwâ Press.

www.ingramcontent.com/pod-product-compliance
Lightning Source LLC
LaVergne TN
LVHW022304200926
848481LV00004B/1215
9798232416393